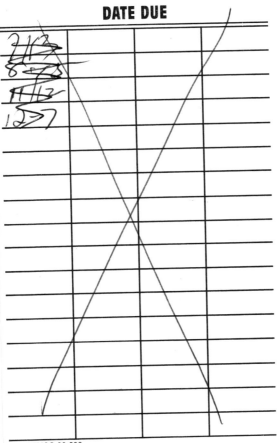

DATE DUE

DEMCO 38-296

Hands of
My Father

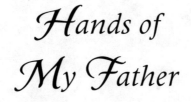

Also by Myron Uhlberg

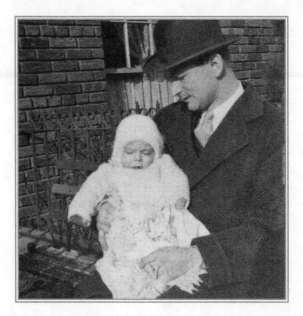

Hands of
My Father

A Hearing Boy, His Deaf Parents,
and the Language of Love

Myron Uhlberg

Bantam Books

HANDS OF MY FATHER
A Bantam Book / February 2009

Published by Bantam Dell
A Division of Random House, Inc.
New York, New York

Book design by Virginia Norey

Bantam Books is a registered trademark of Random House, Inc.,
and the colophon is a trademark of Random House, Inc.

Library of Congress Cataloging-in-Publication Data
Uhlberg, Myron.
Hands of my father : a hearing boy, his deaf parents, and the language
of love / Myron Uhlberg.
p. cm.
ISBN 978-0-553-80688-5 (hardcover)
1. Uhlberg, Myron.   2. Children of deaf parents—United States—Biography.
3. Deaf parents—United States—Biography.   4. Deaf—Family relationships—
United States—Case studies.   I. Title.

HQ759.912U45 2009
306.874092—dc22
[B] 2008025628

Printed in the United States of America
Published simultaneously in Canada

www.bantamdell.com

BVG   10 9 8 7 6 5 4 3 2 1

To the memory of my parents

Louis Uhlberg
1902–1975

Sarah Uhlberg
1906–2001

Author's Note

My parents were deaf, and spoke with their hands, employing signs rather than spoken words to communicate. Today, their language is known as ASL (American Sign Language). Being faithful to the time period of this story, I refer to their language as "sign" and not "Sign." Further, I refer to them as being deaf, the physical condition, as opposed to the conventional "Deaf," used today to indicate the full complexity of Deaf culture.

Finally, as ASL is a visual-gestural language, I have transliterated their conversations from ASL to English. Those conversations, spoken some sixty to seventy years ago—conventionally represented in quotation marks—are not meant to be a word-for-word rendition of what was said, but are, rather, the essence of what was meant.

I have also changed some names in my account.

Gore Vidal observed, in his excellent memoir, *Palimpsest,* "A memoir is how one remembers one's own life." He then went on to say, ". . . even an idling memory is apt to get right what matters most." This memoir is how I remember my life growing up with my deaf parents, and to the best of my ability I've made every effort to get right what matters most. They deserve no less from me, their son.

Acknowledgments

This book would not have been possible without the help of many people.

To Susan Schulman, my agent and friend who suggested that I write this book, and when I had done so, said, "I always place a book that I love." And she did.

To Emily Uhry, whose encouragement and advice in the earliest stages helped shape this book.

To Beth Rashbaum, my editor, who saw in my manuscript a possible book, and then with unlimited patience, goodwill, superb advice, and a firm hand, transformed a disjointed manuscript into the book you now hold in your hand. I owe you more than I can say.

And to her assistant, Angela Polidoro, for her blazingly quick responses to my every question.

Special thanks also to Virginia Norey for her heartfelt design of this book.

To Sue Tarsky, dear old friend who, after a long absence, reentered my life in time to suggest that I could have a second (even a third) career as a writer; and then went out and promptly sold my first two children's books. You changed my life.

To Margaret Quinlin, dear friend, kind soul, dispenser of wisdom in all things literary and beyond, who from the very beginning validated me as a writer.

To Ellen W. Leroe, Eleanor Garner, Milly Lee ("elder sister"), Adrian Fogelin, and, most especially, to Bob and Sandy Weintraub, all writers and staunch friends, to whom I turn for suggestions, advice, and encouragement.

To Sandra Yoon and Pat Lindsay, for their kindness; to Helen Foster Harris for her earliest support; and to Nancy Fritzal, my favorite librarian.

To my fellow CODAs (Children of Deaf Adults), and good friends, Tom Bull, Joyce Linden, and Allyne Bettancourt, for sharing your stories about growing up hearing with deaf parents, and for giving me the encouragement at every step of the way to tell my own story. And to all my CODA brothers and sisters, I respect you and love you all.

To my Brandeis Band of Brothers, almost sixty years and counting, Eddie Manganiello, Charlie Herman, Dick Baldacci, Leo Surette, Jim Stehlin, Bill Orman, Larry Glazer, Tommy Egan, Ron Ranier, Mike Long, Pat Sirkus, Roger Morgan, Dick Bergel, Dave Burman, Ray Deveaux, Rudy Finderson, Mel Nash, and in memory, Hank Thunhorst, Phil Goldstein, Charlie Napoli, Morry Stein, and Jack Kirkwood.

To Joe "Big Red" O'Connor, who listened with sympathy and patience to a problem I had encountered in the writing of this book, and then calmly suggested how I might solve it.

To the best friends a man could ever wish for, Bill McKenna, and in blessed memory, Bob Domozych and Dick Collins, who first met my parents when we were just boys at Brandeis, and who over the years constantly assured me that a book about them would find readers.

To my friends in the Deaf education community, Michelle Gennaoui, Jennifer Storey, and Nancy Boone, who told me as I was writing this book that this was a story that should be told.

To my football coaches: Harry Ostro, at Lafayette High School; Irv Heller, at Brandeis University, and in loving memory of Benny Friedman, two-time college All-American, enshrined in the Pro Football Hall of Fame, and the first athletic director and only football coach at Brandeis University, and his beloved assistant, Harry Stein. I met them as a boy, and they showed me the way to become a man.

To Cindy Bowman, for her friendship, uncritical support, and for showing me what real courage looks like.

To my Brooklyn friends Lenny Lefkowitz, Tommy La Spada, Vico Confino, and in memory, Sam Mark, whom I called incessantly when I was writing about our Brooklyn childhood, checking my memories against theirs.

To Larry Ohrbach and Robert Sax, dear friends who supported me every step of the way in the writing of this book. And special appreciation for the friendship and sound advice of my oldest of friends, Eva and Sam Beller, and George and Sally McGlinnen.

This memoir owes much to my uncle, Milton Wolff, who in the years before his death shared with me his memories—and regrets—about growing up with his deaf sister, Sarah.

To Susan Wolff, daughter of my uncle Milton Wolff, who shared her memories of her complicated father as well as those of our equally complicated grandmother, Celia; and to Jerry Posner, and David and Roberta Trager, who did the same for their parents, my father's younger sisters; and in memory of my cousin, Irving Posner, who would tell me his stories about our grandparents, David and Rebecca.

To my children, Eric, Robin, and Ken, who loved their deaf grandparents, and of whom I am so proud; and to my granddaughters, Alex and Kelli, and my grandsons, Max and Miles, who will one day read this book, and understand.

I am especially grateful to my brother, Irwin, with whom I consulted throughout the writing of this memoir, for his willingness to share with me his memories as well as his deepest feelings about growing up with our deaf parents.

And, as always, to my amazing wife, Karen, my best friend, my first reader, and most trusted advisor in all things literary and otherwise, who at every turn in my life said, "Why not?" You read every chapter, and then, knowing and loving my parents as you did, you told me, with unfailing honesty, and in as few words as possible, whether I had done their story justice. For this, as well as for more than I can say, I am forever grateful to you.

Contents

"What was silent in the father speaks in the son,
and I have often found in the son the
unveiled secret of the father."

—*Friedrich Nietzsche*

Hands of
My Father

Prologue

In the language of the deaf, the sign for *remember* begins with the sign for *know*: the fingertips of the right hand touch the forehead.

But merely to know is not enough, so the sign for *remain* follows: the thumbs of each hand touch and, in this joined position, move steadily forward, into the future. Thus a knowing that remains, never lost, forever: memory.

In my memory, what I remember most vividly are the hands of my father.

My father spoke with his hands. He was deaf. His voice was in his hands.

And his hands contained his memories.

1

The Sound of Silence

My first language was sign.

I was born shortly after midnight, July 1, 1933, my parents' first child. Thus I had one tiny reluctant foot in the first half of that historically fateful year, and the other firmly planted in the second half. In a way my birth date, squarely astride the calendar year, was a metaphor for my subsequent life, one foot always being dragged back to the deaf world, the silent world of my father and of my mother, from whose womb I had just emerged, and the other trying to stride forward into the greater world of the hearing, to escape into the world destined to be my own.

Many years later I realized what a great expression of optimism it was for my father and mother, two deaf people, to decide to have a child at the absolute bottom of the Great Depression.

We lived in Brooklyn, near Coney Island, where on certain summer days, when the wind was blowing just right and our kitchen window was open and the shade drawn up on its roller, I could smell the briny odor of the ocean, layered with just the barest hint of mustard and grilled hot dogs (although that could have been my imagination).

Our apartment was four rooms on the third floor of a new red-brick building encrusted with bright orange fire escapes, which my father and mother had found by walking the neighborhood, and then negotiated for with the impatient hearing landlord all by themselves despite their respective parents' objections that they "could not manage alone" as they were "deaf and handicapped" and "helpless" and would surely "be cheated." They had just returned from their honeymoon, spent blissfully in Washington, D.C., planned to coincide with the silent, colorful explosion of the blossoming cherry trees, which my mother considered a propitious omen for the successful marriage of two deaf people.

Apartment 3A was the only home my father ever knew as a married man. Its four rooms were the place he lived with and loved his deaf wife, and raised his two hearing sons, and then left by ambulance one day forty-four years after arriving there, never to return.

One day my father's hands signed in sorrow and regret the story of how he had become deaf. This was a story he had pieced together from facts he had learned later in life from his younger sister, Rose, who in turn had heard it from their mother. (The fact that he had to learn the details of his own deafness from his younger hearing sister was a source of enduring resentment.)

My father told me he had been born in 1902, a normal hearing child, but at an early age had contracted spinal meningitis. His parents, David and Rebecca, newly arrived in America from Russia, living in an apartment in the Bronx, thought their baby would die.

My father's fever ravaged his little body for over a week. Cold baths during the day and wet sheet–shrouded nights kept him alive. When his fever at last abated, he was deaf. My father would never again hear a sound in all the remaining years of his life. As an adult, he often questioned why it was that he had been singled out as the only member of his family to become deaf.

I, his hearing son, watched his hands sign his anguish: "*Not fair!*"

My father and his father could barely communicate with each other. Their entire shared vocabulary consisted of a few mimed signs: *eat, be quiet, sleep.* These were all command signs. They had no sign for love between them, and his father died without ever having had a single meaningful conversation with his firstborn child.

My father's mother did have a sign for *love.* It was a homemade sign, and she would use it often. My father told me that his language with his mother was poor in quantity but rich in content. She communicated less through agreed-upon signs than through the luminosity that appeared in her eyes whenever she looked at him. That look was special and reserved for him alone.

Like their parents, my father's siblings—his younger brother, Leon, and his two younger sisters, Rose and Millie—never learned a word of formal sign. They remained strangers to him his entire life. At my father's graveside Leon screamed his name, as if, finally, his dead deaf brother had been granted the power to hear his name on his brother's lips.

In 1910, when he was eight years old, my father's parents sent him to live at the Fanwood School for the Deaf, a military-style school for deaf children. My father thought they had abandoned him because he was damaged. In his early days there he cried himself to sleep every night. But ever so slowly he came to realize that rather than having been abandoned, he had been rescued. For the first time in his life he was surrounded by children just like him, and he finally understood that he was not alone in this world.

However, the education he received at Fanwood was certainly a mixed blessing. There, as at most deaf schools at the time, deaf children were taught mainly by hearing teachers, whose goal was to teach them oral speech. The deaf are not mute; they have vocal cords and can speak. But since they cannot monitor the sound of their voice, teaching them intelligible speech is extraordinarily difficult. Although my father and his classmates tried to cooperate with their teachers, not one of them ever learned to speak well enough to be understood by the average hearing person.

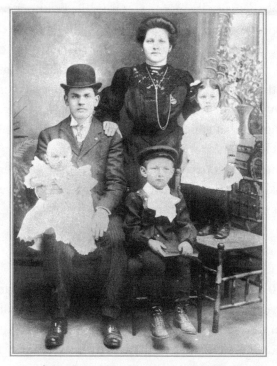

My father, his parents, his sister Rose, and his baby brother, Leon, circa 1907

While this futile and much-resented pedagogic exercise was being inflicted on the deaf children, sign language was strictly forbidden. The hearing teachers considered it to be a primitive method of communication suitable only for the unintelligent.

Not until the 1960s would linguists decree ASL (American Sign Language) to be a legitimate language all its own. But long before then the deaf, among them the children at my father's school, had come to that conclusion themselves. Every night, in the dormitory at Fanwood, the older deaf children taught the younger ones the visual language of sign.

With sign, the boundaries of my father's silent mental universe disappeared, and in the resulting opening sign after new sign accumulated, expanding the closed space within his mind until it filled to bursting with joyous understanding.

"When I was a boy, I was sent to deaf school. I had no real signs," my father signed to me, his hands moving, remembering. "I had only made-up home signs. These were like shadows on a wall. They had no real meaning. In deaf school I was hungry for sign. All were new for me. Sign was the food that fed me. Food for the eye. Food for the mind. I swallowed each new sign to make it mine."

My father's need to communicate was insatiable and would cease only when the dormitory lights were turned out at night. Even then, my father told me, he would sign himself to sleep. Once asleep, my father claimed, he would dream in sign.

My father was taught the printing trade in deaf school, an ideal trade, it was thought, for a deaf man, as printing was a painfully loud business. The unspoken message transmitted to the deaf children of that time by their hearing teachers was that they were neither as smart nor as capable as hearing children. Thus they would primarily be taught manual skills, like printing, shoe repair, and house painting.

Upon graduation in 1920, my father was able to land his first job, the job that would last his working lifetime.

"In the Great Depression," he told me, "I was lucky to have an apprentice job with the *New York Daily News*. I knew it was because I was deaf and so wouldn't be distracted by the noise of the printing presses, and the clattering of the linotype machines, but I didn't care. I also didn't care that the deaf workers were paid less than the hearing workers because Captain Patterson, the big boss, knew that we wouldn't, couldn't, complain. He knew that we would be happy for any job, at any wage. We were deaf. He could hear. And he was right. The hearing people ran the world.

"But those were tough times for me. By the time I gave my mother money out of my small pay envelope at the end of the week, for my room and board, and then some more for the household expenses, there was not much left over. My hearing brother and sisters did not have steady work. My mother and father were the janitors of our building, so they had little ready cash. It broke my heart to see my mother on her hands and knees, shuffling up and down the hallways, washing the wooden floors with hot, soapy water she dragged along behind her in a big wooden bucket. Her hands were always red and raw. To this day I can't get the memory of her chafed hands out of my mind. When I finally got my union card and made good union wages, I could give her enough money every month so she didn't have to do that anymore. You can't imagine how proud I was that I, her deaf son, could do that for her."

As an apprentice, he explained to me, he worked the night shift. It was known as the "lobster shift," for no reason that he was ever able to explain to me. As a boy, I reasoned that since he worked nights while everyone else was asleep, including fish in the ocean, it must be that lobsters were awake during those hours, and hence the name.

Being a printer was the only job my father ever had, and he loved it. He would work for the newspaper until he retired over forty years later. In all that time he worked side by side with hearing co-workers, but he never really knew them. Like most in the hearing world, they treated him as if he were an alien—primitive, incapable of speech, and lacking human thought: a person to be avoided if possible, and if not, ignored.

After an apprenticeship of many years, my father was issued a union card. It was the proudest moment of his life. It was tangible proof that he was as good as any hearing man. Even in the dark days of the Depression, when one out of four men were out of work, he, a deaf man, could support himself.

And, he reasoned, he could also support a wife. My father was tired of being alone in this hearing world. It was time, he thought, to create his own silent world. A world that would begin with a deaf wife.

One bleak winter day, while we were sitting at the kitchen table, the rain sleeting against the windows of our Brooklyn apartment, his hands told me the rest of his story, in which began my story:

"Sarah was a young girl. She had many friends. She liked to have fun.

"I first noticed her at the beach in Coney Island. She was always laughing.

"All the deaf boys were crazy about Sarah. Even the hearing boys.

"There were many handsome boys on the beach. All the young boys had muscles and chocolate tans. They could jump and leap over each other's backs. They could do handstands.

"I was older. I didn't have muscles. I couldn't stand on my hands if my life depended on it. I didn't have a brown tan. I would get sunburned. My skin turned red. And then I would peel.

"It didn't matter. The handsome young boys with their chocolate skin and big muscles only wanted to have fun with Sarah. They were not serious boys. They had no jobs. So they had plenty of time to play, and make muscles, and get brown skin from the sun.

"I was a serious man. I had a job. A good job. The best job. I was no longer an apprentice printer. I had a union card, just like the hearing workers.

"I didn't want Sarah just to have fun. I wanted a wife for all time. I wanted a mother for my children. I wanted a partner forever. We would be two deaf people in the hearing world. We would make our own world. A quiet world. A silent world.

"We would be strong together, and strong for our children."

Then, just as the rain stopped and thin rays of sunlight striped the tabletop, my father smiled to himself, his hands thinking . . .

"Maybe we would have a little fun before the children came."

Lost in reverie, his hands, bathed in golden light, now lay silent on the kitchen table. Time passed. I sat and watched his still hands, waiting patiently for them to continue his story. I loved the quiet time we spent together, and I loved the stories his hands contained.

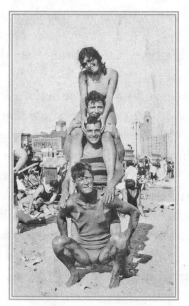

*My mother at
Coney Island*

Then my father's hands came alive again, eloquently describing a warm spring afternoon in 1932 Brooklyn.

"I knew I had to make a good impression.

"I had to dress well. I wore my best suit. Actually, it was my only suit. The big Depression was still going strong, and I watched every dollar."

He tells me his suit was a fine wool serge that cost him two weeks' salary. Its jaunty design was at odds with the feeling of dread that grew in him that day as he set off for the apartment where Sarah lived with her family, having written to her father asking if he might pay a call.

The scene unfolds with cinematic vividness as my father's hands recount each stage of his quest.

He descends with the crowd, down the stairs from the subway platform, sweat dampening his armpits, and exits the station into the frantic gay activity of Sabbath shoppers rushing about, making their last-minute purchases for the evening meal.

The salt scent of the Atlantic Ocean hangs over every shop awning, every outdoor stall, reminding my father, as if he needed such a reminder, how far he had traveled this warm day from his familiar home in the northern leafy village reaches of the Bronx, after one trolley ride and three subway transfers, to the very end of Brooklyn, on the honky-tonk shore of Coney Island. And why has he come here on this warm spring day, sweat pooling at the base of his spine, palms moistly clutching now-wilted store-bought flowers? Today, this very afternoon, my father will meet, for the first time, the family of the girl he has chosen to be his wife.

Unfortunately for him, my future mother, waiting at home, believes he is hopelessly boring and much too old for her; besides, she feels, she's too young to be married, there being so much fun to be had with all the good-looking boys who flutter around her like bees around a hive of honey every weekend on the hot sand of Bay 6, their hands gesturing wildly to gain her exclusive attention. And she could not banish from her mind the image of the hearing golden boy whose attentions she enjoyed so much and who said he loved her.

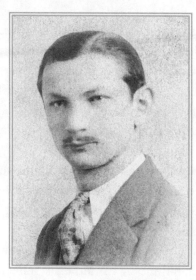

My father, circa 1932

Glancing nervously at the written directions, my father marches down the broad bustling avenue, so unlike the uneventful Bronx street where he lives. His hands at his sides rehearse the arguments he will employ this afternoon to convince this dark-haired young girl and her father that he is the one to whom she should commit her future. He has been marshaling the arguments in his favor for the past two weeks. He has a steady job and a union card. He is mature and serious. He is a loyal and dependable fellow, calm in an emergency. He can read. He can write. He can sign fluently. And if she will have him, he will love her forever. He finds himself impressed with his qualifications as he cycles through them. He is an up-and-comer. Besides, he has a full head of hair parted perfectly down the middle and a dandy mustache, and is altogether a fine-looking fellow.

Fifteen crowded blocks from the subway station, on a narrow tree-lined side street, he finds her apartment building, fronted with a narrow stoop, a five-story walkup in a typical dumbbell front-to-back floor arrangement.

Up goes my father. Up the stone steps of the stoop. Up the five flights of spongy wooden stairs. Up through the hallway smells of cooking and laundry and close immigrant living. Arriving at the door of 5B, he pauses. His future lies behind the dark wooden door. He thinks: What if her parents don't like him? What if they disapprove of him? What if they think he is too deaf? What will he do if they don't give their blessings to his cause? How will he endure if he cannot have this magnificent girl for his wife? He'll do anything, he thinks, to win their approval. He'll even move to Brooklyn, if that is the price he must pay to be accepted.

He knocks. The door opens, and he is greeted by a compact, tightly coiled, unsmiling man in mismatched jacket and pants who waves at him, making clumsy unintelligible signs with his large paint-stained hands. My father does not understand a word he is saying but reasons that this is a greeting of sorts, and an invitation to enter the apartment.

My father enters and in a single glance takes in the entirety of the apartment. From front to back, cheek to jowl, it is filled with large, mismatched pieces of heavy dark wood furniture buffed to a high shine. There seems to be at least two of everything, leaving barely space to move about. My father thinks this apartment looks more like a furniture shop on the Lower East Side than a living space. Unbeknownst to him, my mother's father had rented all this furniture and arranged for it to be delivered just that morning with the thought of impressing him, the suitor of his daughter. My father is not impressed. He is confused.

My mother sits at one of the two dining room tables, and as my father signs his excited greeting to her, she bursts into tears. On the two couches, staring expressionlessly at my father, sit the family: mother, three sons, and another daughter.

Confused by the abundance of furniture, the stony looks of the family, and the tears of my mother, my father wonders what he has gotten himself into. He finally seats himself in one of the twelve chairs surrounding the two dining room tables, facing the family.

At once, as if in a coin-operated game at Coney Island, the frozen tableau comes to life, and all the members of my mother's family break into excited gestures and frantic hand- and arm-waving. They are trying to put my father at ease, but their home-made signs are virtual Greek to his eyes. Perhaps, my father thinks, this is a Brooklyn accent.

My father smiles politely and occasionally nods in agreement at what he thinks is the appropriate time.

My mother wipes her tears away, and for the first time since her father opened the front door, she smiles a shy tentative smile. All doubt and confusion depart from my father's mind. He addresses her father and begins to make his case in simple sign language and written notes. My mother's father does not understand a word my father is saying. He does not understand the signs. Must be a Bronx accent, he thinks. And my father's notes are largely incomprehensible to him.

Nonetheless he smiles from time to time behind his shaggy gray beard, nodding in tune with my father's broad gestures. Emboldened by the seeming agreement, my father grows more expansive in his signs, describing his position as a printer at the *New York Daily News,* "lobster shift" to be sure, but daytime work just around the corner now that he has his union card.

My mother translates what my father says in their homemade signs. Now her father smiles broadly and nods energetically. He feels confident that this serious young deaf man really is the answer to his prayers. This is someone who is from his daughter's world, someone who will be able to take care of her.

My father has no more to say. He has made his case to the girl's father. But what of the girl?

My father asks her father if he can take his daughter out for the rest of the afternoon. Perhaps a walk on the boardwalk. *"Yes, yes, by all means,"* the bearded face nods in agreement.

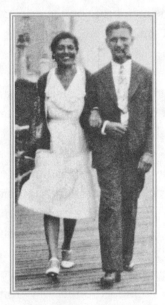

My mother and father on the boardwalk at Coney Island

My father and this beautiful girl walk on the boardwalk from Coney Island to Brighton Beach, then back again to the starting point. Although the girl has gone to the Lexington School for the Deaf and is as fluent in sign language as my father, they have said very little to each other. Now they rest on a bench and look at the waves rolling in, one after the other, with great interest, while their hands sit quietly in their laps.

As the light fades from the sky over Coney Island, signaling the beginning of the end of this momentous day, my father takes my mother's hand in his strong printer's hands and gently squeezes her fingers. She returns the pressure with a slight acknowledging squeeze of her own.

One week later three strong young men climb five flights of wooden stairs and quickly remove all the splendid two-of-everything rented furniture. Rented by the day, it has served its purpose, now that my father has proposed and Sarah has accepted. On the return trip the men bring up the original shabby, mismatched pieces—which come in ones, not twos.

Shortly thereafter Louis and Sarah were married. Barely nine months after the wedding, at the height of a thunderstorm, I was born in Coney Island Hospital.

My father's hands described what that frightful day had been like. His hands appeared to be warding off something. Something unknown that caused fear. "It was a dreadful day," he signed, throwing out his hands from alongside his temples. *"Awful!"*

It was the hottest day of the summer. All of Brooklyn lay stunned beneath the heat. The angry sun had baked the sands of Coney Island and turned the blue Atlantic into a sea of molten red. At dusk the boiling sun continued on its way from Brooklyn to California, taking with it the light but leaving behind the heat.

My father's hands told me how he paced the grimy linoleum floor of the hospital. From end to end in the airless hallway he measured off his steps: one hundred one way, one hundred back again. And with each step he signed to himself his frustration and his fear.

Back and forth, back and forth, past his wife's room, past the weeping walls, he walked his endless circle of anxiety. He had been doing this for ten hours, ever since his wife had been admitted after her waters broke so shockingly, signaling the impending birth of their first child.

My father had no thought for the child who was taking his time to arrive, only for his wife, lying on sweat-drenched sheets, in a room he was not permitted to enter, from which few if any news bulletins came his way.

Some time after the sun set a cold front suddenly moved in over Brooklyn, bringing with it a drop of forty degrees in temperature. The cold air rear-ended the darkening boiling mass in its path. Lightning split the sky, and rain fell in cold torrents onto the steaming asphalt streets of Coney Island. Day turned to darkest night.

Soon the tar-topped street outside the hospital was filled from curb to curb with the rising tide of water. The sewers could not handle the overflow, and the water backed up, rising quickly above the hubcaps of the parked cars, flowing down neighboring cellar steps. The violent electric storm spawned winds that toppled trees and tore down telephone poles, while five floors above my father continued his solitary pacing, wondering how he could possibly exist in a world without his deaf wife, Sarah.

Lightning struck oil tanks in New Jersey, sending flames hundreds of feet into the sky, turning night back into blazing day; and the wind tore down a circus tent in Queens, trapping four hundred people beneath the rain-drenched canvas. All the windows of Brooklyn went dark as power lines fell like matchsticks, and my father became a father.

"I rushed out into the storm raising my fist to the heavens," his hands told me. "I was a crazy man. A Niagara of water submerged me, and all about bolts of lightning splintered the sky."

Over the crashing sounds of this Olympian tumult, my father's deaf voice cried out, *"God, make my son hear!"*

*   *   *

*C*ould I hear? That was the question. The answer was, he didn't know.

"But," his hands continued, "we were determined to find out. And quickly!"

The reason for the doubt on my father's part was that he and his family had no sure way of knowing the reason for his own deafness. Yes, they all agreed, my father had been quite sick as a young boy; he had run a high fever and, when better, was discovered to have lost all hearing. The same was the case with my mother, who, it was thought, had scarlet fever when just a baby.

But, their parents reasoned, the illness and the deafness were not necessarily connected. Their many other children had also been sick at one time or another, and they had also had high fevers, but they were not deaf. They did not have "broken ears."

"Both sets of parents were dead set against our having children," my father signed. "They thought a child of ours would be born deaf. They were ignorant immigrants from the old country." His hands beat the air angrily. "What the hell did they know? Anyway, they treated us like children. Always. Even when we were adults ourselves. They couldn't help it. We were deaf, and so we were helpless in their minds. Like children. We would always be children to them. So we did not listen to them, and we had you. They were surprised when they saw how perfect you were. Nothing missing. A regular baby. A *normal* baby in their eyes.

"Mother Sarah and I loved you from the first time we saw you. But secretly some part of us wished you were born deaf."

Although I loved my father and mother, I could not imagine being part of their deaf world. And I could not understand why even the smallest secret part of them could wish such a fate for me.

"You were our first child," his hands explained. "We were deaf in a hearing world. There was no one to tell us how to raise a hearing child. We did not have the hearing language to ask. And hearing people did not have our language to tell us. We were on our own. Always. There was no one to help us. How were we to know what you wanted, what you needed? How were we to know when you cried in the dark? When you were hungry? Happy? Sad? When you had a pain in your stomach?

"And how," he said, "would we tell you we loved you?"

My father paused. His hands were still, thoughtful.

"I was afraid I would not know you if you were a hearing baby. I feared you would not know your deaf father."

Then he smiled. "Mother Sarah was not worried. She said she

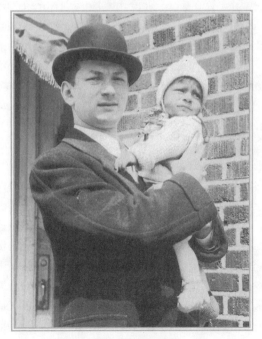

My father and I

was your mother. She would know you. She said you were the son from her body, and you would know your mother. There was no need for mouth-speak. No need for hand-speak.

"When we brought you home from the hospital, we arranged for Mother Sarah's family to come to our apartment every Saturday afternoon. 'Urgent!' I wrote. 'You must come! Every week. Saturday.'

"They listened. They came from Coney Island every Saturday for all of your first year of life. They never missed, all of them: Mother Sarah's mother and father, and her younger sister and three younger brothers. They ate like horses, but it was worth it."

"How boring that must have been for them," I signed, pressing my finger to my nose as if to a grindstone wheel.

"We didn't care. I had a plan," he signed vigorously. "They always came when you were sleeping. I made sure of that. Before making themselves comfortable, I asked them to stand at the back of your crib. Then they pounded on pots and pans I gave them. You heard a big noise and snapped awake, and you began to wail. It was a wonderful sight to see you cry so strongly at the heavy noise sound."

"Wonderful?" I asked. "Wonderful for who? Now I know why I have trouble sleeping some nights."

My father continued, ignoring my complaint.

"We celebrated. Mother Sarah served them tea and honey cake. When no one was looking, your Hungarian grandfather, Max the Gypsy, slipped booze into his tea from a silver flask he carried. As he sipped his tea, he would add another shot. Soon his teacup was filled just with whiskey, and he would sip and smile, smile and sip, all afternoon long. 'Ah, thank God, Myron can hear,' he would mumble, as he took another sip. Your grandmother, Celia, would look at him in her tight-lipped way, like he was a cockroach she had surprised when turning on the kitchen light late at night. She always looked like she wanted to step on him. No one seemed to notice this, but we deaf see everything. I see more meaning in one blink of an eye than my hearing brother and sisters hear in an hour-long conversation. They understand nothing. The mouth speaks words they hear but teach them nothing. I love my brother and sisters but they are not as smart as me.

"No matter, that's not part of your hearing story. That's another story."

My father's memories were so intense, and so tightly woven together in his mind, that in the midst of telling one story, he would often wander off into another one that rose to the surface almost as if it had been bottled up all these years and, now that there was someone to tell it to, had just worked itself free. When he did so, he would catch himself and terminate the beginning of the new memory by abruptly signing *another story*. And then I knew that, somewhere down the road, I would hear from him this *other story*.

"On Sundays my mother, father, brother, and two sisters came down from the Bronx. They did not trust Mother Sarah's family. They brought their own pots and pans. Each one held a pot or a pan on their lap during the two-hour, three-subway-ride trip from way up in the Bronx to Kings Highway in Brooklyn. They practiced banging on the pots and pans while the subway cars went careening through the tunnels. The train's wheels made such a screeching sound that people on the car barely noticed them. When they got off the subway, my sisters and brother marched to our apartment house, still banging the pots and pans. They looked like some ragtag army in a Revolutionary War painting. As soon as they arrived at our apartment, they hid behind the head of your bed and pounded away, while they stomped their feet like a marching band. I felt the loud noise through the soles of my feet. They had a nice rhythm. The result was the same: you awoke immediately. Jumped, actually."

"This went on for a whole *year?*" I asked.

"Yes. They thought your hearing might go away. Just as hearing for me and Mother Sarah went away when we were young. Big mystery."

"How about our neighbors? All that banging and stomping, didn't they mind?" I asked.

"What do you expect?" my father answered. "We had to know if your hearing stayed with you. The neighbors threatened to call the landlord. Have us evicted. Mother Sarah sweet-talked them out of it. The notes flew fast and furious between them till they settled down. Anyway, they thought you were a cute baby. They also wondered if you could hear. They wondered if the deaf can have a hearing baby. We were the only deaf people they knew. They had no idea of our deaf ways."

Thinking for a minute, his hands added, striking each other sharply, "It was *hard* for Mother Sarah and me to figure out how to take care of you. But we did. We learned how to tell when you cried at night. You slept in your crib next to our bed when we brought you home from the hospital. We kept a small light on all night. Mother Sarah wore a ribbon attached to her wrist and to your sweet baby foot. When you moved your foot, she would immediately awaken to see the reason why. She still has that ribbon somewhere. Sign was your first language. The first sign you learned was *I love you.*

"That is a good sign. The best sign."

Memorabilia

A Fox in Brooklyn

Memory unwinds, like the steel spring of a windup clock.

I see myself as a small child, still so young that I am sleeping in my parents' bedroom. I'm dressed in feet-pajamas that sport a practical drop-down seat flap. It is night. Something wakes me. So I go to wake my father. My hand on his shoulder was my first form of communication: touch. Soon after touch came sign, another language of hands.

"What?" He jerks upright at the insistent shaking of his shoulder, simultaneously signing to me: his upturned hands wiggle imploringly, back and forth, demanding an answer. His face is a mask of puzzlement and inquiry. His shoulders hunch up in expectation of an answer. *What?* his long-drawn-out sign demands. Since he is deaf, and I can hear, he cannot permit any misunderstanding between us.

What? was one of the earliest signs I remember acquiring. Almost every exchange between my deaf father and me began with the sign for *What?* My answer would decode many things for him. My needs. My feelings. My emotions. My state of mind. My request for information.

Virtually all communication between us took off from my response to that question: *What?* With this essential foundational exchange accomplished, he was able to proceed appropriately.

On this night, at midnight, the "what" was my fear.

"I heard a noise," I signed, pointing to my ear and banging

my small fists together. Since I was scared of the noise, my fists beat a strong tattoo against each other. My father stilled my hands and got out of bed.

"Show me," he signed.

I think back on that exchange between my father and me so very long ago and realize that it must have been the first time I realized my father was deaf.

How could I *show* him the sound?

I took his hand in mine and pointed it to the closet. That's where the sound was coming from.

As I clung to his leg, he opened the closet door. There, from the darkness, staring down at me, was the furry face of a fox, its bright unblinking eyes looking straight into mine, its small pointy ears taking in the sound of my choked, whimpering sobs. I looked back through half-closed wet eyelids, squinting in reflexive fear, as I saw the fox hunching his shoulders, preparing to spring at me. His gaping narrow mouth was filled with hundreds of small white pointy teeth. I could feel those teeth shredding my arm.

I screamed for my mother, but my mother slept on, her back turned to the sight of her only child about to be eaten alive. *Doesn't she care?* My young mind could not process the fact that she could not hear the fox's snarling, hungry anticipation of biting down on her son's soft fleshy arm.

With his hands my father grabbed the fox by the neck and yanked him from his perch. Shaking the fox back and forth, he squeezed the life out of him. Now the eyes of the fox turned glassy, all life drained away. The fox hung limply, tail down, lifeless, in my father's strong hands. Hands that gently held me, stroked my head, hugged me, and spoke to me. "Don't be afraid. The fox won't bother you anymore."

Throwing the dead fox on the floor of the closet, he

slammed the door on my nightmare, wiped the tears from my eyes, and led me back to my bed. As he tucked me tightly under my quilt, he looked at me for the longest time, a half-smile on his lips. Then, holding my face in his hands, he softly kissed me. And I went to sleep.

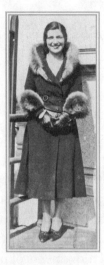

*My mother and
her fox stole*

This recollection was for a long time a sharp pebble on the far shore of memory. From time to time, as I walked the beach of my childhood memories, I would step, barefooted, on that particular pebble. What exactly was that fearsome creature lurking in the closet that so infected my dreams? Surely there were no wild foxes running around in Brooklyn. At least not on my block; not in my apartment; and certainly not in my parents' closet.

Many years later I realized that the monster my father killed for me that night must have been my mother's fox-fur stole.

2

The Child as Father of the Man

My second language was spoken English.

I have no memory of learning this language, or at what age, but somehow I did. And with the acquisition of spoken language, a big part of my childhood ended before it began. As the hearing child of a deaf father, I was expected to perform the daily alchemy of transmuting the silent visual movements of my father's hands into the sound of speech and meaning for the hearing, and then to perform the magic all over again for him, in reverse, transmuting invisible sound into visible sign.

Many years later, as a student in college, I came across this line from Wordsworth: "The child is father of the man." I immediately understood its meaning—even if it wasn't what Wordsworth himself had intended.

At times while acting as my father's human conduit between sign and sound, I felt not unlike the telephone wires strung from pole to pole down the backyards of our Brooklyn neighborhood: wires through which compressed sound was somehow magically converted and transported, to emerge at the other end as comprehensible speech. As a deaf family, we had no telephone. I was our human telephone, lacking only a dial tone, but like a telephone I was available for instant use at all hours of the day or night, completely at the whim and needs of its owner, my deaf father.

In addition to playing this role, I also found myself increasingly called upon to explain sound to my father, as if sound were a tangible thing that, although invisible, if explained properly, comprehensively, even exhaustively by me, could be imagined by my deaf father and thus, with understanding, made real for him.

For as long as I can remember, I always had a radio. Just as I cannot disassociate memories of my existence in my crib from the discordant sound of banging pots and pans, so too there was always music, and the music of speech. My father had decided shortly after bringing me home from the hospital that sound was something that I would *learn* to hear, and having learned it, I would not lose this ability through disuse. He was convinced, since there was no one to tell him otherwise, that one acquired and maintained the ability to hear by practice. The Philco radio he bought to ensure my constant exposure to sound sat on a small stand by the head of my bed, just beyond the wooden slats of my crib. It was turned on day and night. The yellow light that illuminated the dial was my nightlight. And I was quite comforted both by the warm yellow light and by the sound pouring unceasingly from that wood-and-cloth box. The light and the sound accompanied me to sleep every night.

When I was older and left my crib for a bed with no sides, alongside my new grown-up bed in my very own room was a new grown-up radio. I had graduated from a table-model radio, standing on four little feet, to a solid piece of heavy dark wooden furniture that sat gravely on my bedroom floor. It was taller than me and looked not unlike a cathedral, with an arched dome and a tracery face, like the quatrefoil rose window of Chartres Cathedral, but filled with cloth insets instead of bits of stained glass. Its chunky knobs completely filled my childish hands.

Although I've been asked a thousand times how I learned to speak, I have no clear recollection of the process of acquiring speech, that *eureka!* moment of comprehension. I can't help but think that the radio playing constantly alongside my ear, from a time beyond memory, contributed to my brain's cracking the code of oral speech in my otherwise silent world.

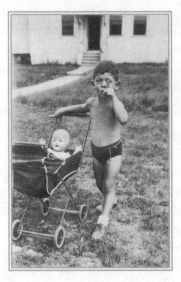

Here I'm pushing a doll in a baby carriage, while signing "girl."

The radio also became the Rosetta Stone for my father's eternal quest in deciphering, and so understanding, sound. Unlike the Rosetta Stone, my radio had no visible symbols that could be, with thought and analysis, converted into language. But it did have the light that lit the dial, a dial with numbers and fractions of numbers, and an arrow that settled from time to time on certain numbers, some more often than others. And then there were the numbers that resided at each extreme end of the dial, numbers upon which the dial never settled.

My father struggled to understand how the radio worked. He removed the back and studied the many tubes of the chassis and noted how they flickered on like candles, wavered, and then burned brightly, steadily.

"Beautiful, but it's not meant for us deaf," his hands informed me, more resigned than sad.

And yet he was fascinated by this mechanism that was both object and process. "Is sound confined to specific sections of time and space? Is there no sound between the numbers?"

The fact that, after the dial light stayed on for a while, the whole affair grew warm to his touch, gave rise to another set of questions.

"Is sound warm?" he asked. "When the radio is cold, is there no sound coming from it? Can there be sound in the Arctic, where it is always cold? Is there sound everywhere down around the equator, where it's hot? Is Africa a noisy place? Alaska quiet?"

When he held his hands, reverentially cupping the smooth mahogany cathedral dome of the radio, he felt rising and falling vibrations sounding off the wood. "Does sound have rhythm? Does it rise and fall like the ocean? Does sound come and go like the wind?" I struggled for years trying to come up with answers for my father, to explain the inexplicable to him.

Although my father could not hear the music coming from my radio, he could feel it through the soles of his feet. When he tired of asking me questions, he would pull my mother to him, and together they would dance to the rhythm of the music rising up from the hardwood floor, whirling in perfect harmony around my bedroom, as smoothly as Fred Astaire and Ginger Rogers.

*   *   *

My father was an adult, I a mere child, but as he could neither hear nor speak comprehensibly in the hearing world outside our silent apartment, I became his designated ears and mouth. This began when I was still a little boy, not more than five or six. One day he took me to the poultry shop at the corner of our block, where the chickens hung from the hooks in the ceiling, their blind eyes looking down at the sawdust-covered floor. My father's hands began to move.

"Tell Mr. Herman we want a fat chicken today," he signed, two fingers moving up and down like the beak of a pecking bird. Some of his signs were so real, they made me laugh. He laughed right along with me and would then exaggerate the sign. Soon everybody around us would be laughing also. When I was older, I realized they had been laughing at us, not with us.

Our next stop was the vegetable stand.

"Mother Sarah loves corn," he signed, his fingers scraping imaginary kernels from an imaginary corncob. "But it must be fresh. Absolutely fresh." My job was to select the yellowest ears with the juiciest kernels, the plumpest of red tomatoes, the heaviest potatoes, and the crispest heads of lettuce.

"Good," he signed, thumbs up. "These are perfect." My father always said that, even the time a fat worm crawled out of a tomato I had selected with such care.

"Only a perfect tomato like this one," he signed, "would attract such a perfect worm."

Out on the street my father's hands told me, "Tomorrow we will go to the zoo."

Magically his hands turned into animals. Slowly they swayed like an elephant's trunk. Fingers curled, they scratched his side like a monkey. Lightly they brushed his nose like a mouse twitching his whiskers. And his thumb peeked out from beneath the shell of his hand like a turtle's head. As I watched, my father's hands shaped the air, and I saw a zoo filled with flying birds, slithering snakes, snapping alligators, and sleek swimming seals.

People stopped and looked at us. I looked only at my father's hands, imagining the fun we would have and the sights we would see.

Walking home, we passed a man sitting on the curb. "I'm hungry," he whispered.

The man was old. His clothes were dirty. I didn't want to stop.

"What did the man say?" my father asked.

"He's hungry," I answered.

My father reached into our paper bags and pulled out some apples and a loaf of bread to give to the man.

"Tell him I'm sorry." With his fist he circled his heart. "But tell him things are bound to get better." Then he took my hand, and we continued down the street.

When we arrived back home, my mother was waiting by our apartment door. My father smiled, put down the paper bags, waved his arms in an excited greeting, and gathered her in his arms. There was room for me as well.

*W*hen I was a small child, interpreting for my father while shopping in the chicken store and vegetable market made me feel important. However, even though my role as interpreter was a source of pride, it often left me feeling confused. Here I was, mouthing the adult words and concepts of my father, an adult, to another adult. But I was not an adult. I was a six-year-old child. And in those bygone times in Brooklyn, the role of a child was quite clear. Children were spoken *to*. They were constantly being told what to do and how to act: "Do this." "Do that." "Come here." "Go there." And most embarrassingly, as if kids were dogs, "*Sit*."

The only order that was missing from parents' lexicon of commands was "Heel."

A kid's life was one of commands. There was no room for discussion between child and parent. Whine? Yes. Up to a point. Discuss? No. Never.

But unlike my friends, who unthinkingly knew their place in the scheme of things, I had a dual role. Their fathers could hear and thus did not depend on them for anything; mine could not. And when he was forced to interact with the hearing, my father was placed in the position of a child—ignored or dismissed. At those times my father expected me to transform myself instantly into an adult, one who was capable of communicating on his behalf, adult to adult.

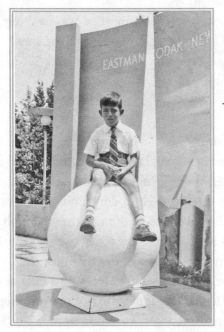

At the 1939 World's Fair, looking very crabby because I've had to translate for my father all day.

Mastering this unique trick of two-way communication—sound to sign, sign to sound—put me in an odd, unnatural position relative to my father. In a complete reversal of normal status, my deaf father was dependent on his hearing child.

Further compounding my confusion, in my guise as presumptive adult I often felt invisible. My father had programmed me to be a mere conduit for communication when I was interpreting for him: he spoke not *to* me but *through* me, like a pane of glass.

Dizzying as all that was, the moment my father did not need my trick, the roles were suddenly flipped around, and once again I was the child.

These polarizing reversals, so sudden and complete, were unnerving for me. One minute I was struggling with comprehending and deciphering, then translating and interpreting the adult concepts that had been communicated to me by hearing grown-ups. The very next minute my father was ordering me to be still, to stop jumping around, and to stop fidgeting—and telling me that a boy must always mind his father. Then he would gently but firmly take my small hand in his, and we would walk away from the hearing world, and I would be once again just what I was, his little boy.

As I grew older, my job as interpreter increased in complexity, and so did my feelings about it. My father continued to take me with him every Saturday morning to do the week's shopping, and I still felt a sense of pride about his reliance on me. But in time I became increasingly sensitive to the harsh reality of the prejudice and scorn that the hearing world levied at my deaf father.

Older still, as I deepened into the role of being my father's voice, I would note with despair and shame, and then anger, the way in which the hearing would ignore him as if he were nothing more than an inanimate, insensate block of stone, something not quite human. This sheer indifference seemed even worse than contempt.

On many occasions I witnessed a hearing stranger approach my father on the street and ask him a question: "Can you tell me the way to the subway?" "What time is it?" "Where is the closest bakery?"

I was never able to get used to the initial look of incomprehension that bloomed on the stranger's face when my father failed to answer, and the way that look turned to shock at the sound of his harsh voice announcing his deafness, then metastasized into revulsion, at which point the stranger would turn and flee as if my father's deafness were a contagious disease.

Even now, seventy long years in the future, the memory of the shame I sometimes felt as a child is as corrosive as battery acid in my veins, and bile rises unbidden in my throat.

One day we were in the local butcher shop. As usual on a Saturday, it was crowded. My father told me to ask the butcher for five pounds of rib roast. "Tell the butcher man, no fat!" he added firmly.

"My father wants five pounds of rib roast. No fat," I said to the butcher when we got to the head of the line.

"I'm busy, kid," he said, not even bothering to look at my father. "Tell him you'll have to wait your turn."

"What did he say?" my father asked me.

"He said we have to wait our turn."

"But it *is* our turn. Tell the man to wait on us. Now!"

"My father says it's our turn now. He would like a five-pound rib roast, and no fat."

I added politely, "Please, mister."

"Tell the *dummy* I'll say when it's his turn. Now get to the back of the line, or get the hell out of my store."

The line of restless shoppers now stood as statues, frozen in their places, staring with blank, unfeeling eyes.

"What did the man say?" my father asked me.

Above all else my father had taught me that I must never, *ever* edit what hearing people directed at him, no matter what they said. He wanted it straight. Thus I signed, *"The man says you're a dummy,"* while a roaring furnace burned within my six-year-old body, almost blistering my skin.

I had never heard anyone call my father a dummy before. The only time I had ever heard the word was on the radio during the Charlie McCarthy show, when Edgar Bergen called Charlie a dummy. "Charlie, you're a dummy. You're nothing but a block of wood."

My father was not a block of wood. He was no dummy.

My father's face flushed with anger.

"Tell the man to shove the roast up his ass!" he signed with exaggerated emphasis.

"My father says we'll be back, thank you."

Outside on the street my father knelt down to me.

"I know you didn't tell the butcher man what I told you," he signed. "I could tell by looking at his face. That's okay. I understand. You were embarrassed.

"It's not fair, I know.

"I'm in the deaf world.

"You're in the hearing world.

"I need you to help me in your world. Hearing people have no time for a deaf man. No time to read my notes. They have no patience for the deaf. Hearing people think I'm stupid. *I am not stupid.*"

My father's hands fell silent.

"No matter what they think," he finally signed to me, "I must still deal with them. So I must ask you for help. You can hear. You can speak."

My father was always so sure of himself. But now he seemed different. And I thought he might cry. I had never seen my father cry. I couldn't even imagine it. And it scared me.

Looking directly into my eyes, he slowly signed, "It hurts me to have this need for you. You're just a boy. I hope you will understand and not hate me."

Hate my father? I was shocked. How could he think that?

"No." I shook my head.

"Never!" my hand said.

My father took me in his arms and kissed me, then held my head to his chest, and I heard his beating heart.

Not long after the butcher shop incident, my grandmother Celia told me, "You must always take care of your parents!" That's all she said. She didn't explain herself, or give me any instructions about how to follow her advice. However, I vividly remember what she told me that day because it was so baffling to me. How could I, a child, take care of them, adults? And not just any adults—they were my mother and father. But I would learn.

Memorabilia

The Language of Touch

From the time I was a small child, I was struck by how often my father would hold me, for no reason that I could ever understand. On my block it was quite noticeable, even to a young kid like me. In that time men had the socially accepted role of breadwinner. They were not the nurturers of our young lives. That role was reserved for our mothers.

Every weekday morning while it was still dark, the apartment houses on our block would empty of all our fathers. The men would march with heavy-lidded eyes, virtually in lockstep, to the subway station on Kings Highway, from which the subway trains would whisk them off to points all over Brooklyn, as well as to "the city." (No Brooklynite *ever* called the *city* "Manhattan.") There our fathers toiled in largely meaningless tasks, uncomplainingly, since the Depression was not far from memory. Latter-day concepts of having a "career" or work that was "fulfilling" would have been Greek to their ears. A "job" plain and simple, the ability to earn that which was sufficient to "put bread on the table" and pay the rent—that's what our fathers' daily tasks in those days were all about.

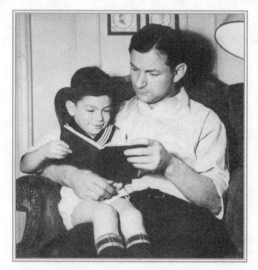

My father and I

At precisely one hour before supper, the fathers of our block would return, shoulders turned downward, heads bent, the *New York Daily News* held tightly under their arms.

The women would proceed to greet their husbands, often launching into a well-documented list of *their* child's misbehavior that very day. This litany of misdeeds might result in a swat on the head to the errant child with the folded *Daily News*—or worse.

On my block, in those long-ago days, this was often the only physical connection a father would make with his son.

But that was not the case with my father. At the end of his workday he would drop to his knees when he saw me, and hold me close, as if I had been lost, then found. After that first embrace he would hold me at arm's length, looking me over long and deeply. On his face I would detect a look of mild surprise, a look I could never decipher. No signs were exchanged between us. All that I needed, in order to understand how much my father loved me, was the feel of his arms around me. He spoke, and the language I heard was the language of his touch.

3
The Fights

My interpreting for my father was an external business. It occurred on the outside, in the hearing world. One day, though, I was called upon to perform my trick inside the walls of our apartment, and this time I was put to a test beyond my calendar years, and many light-years beyond my skills.

It was a June night in 1938, and the occasion was a rematch between Joe Louis, the black man known as America's Brown Bomber, and Max Schmeling, Adolf Hitler's example of presumed Nazi racial superiority, a product of the Master Race. In their first fight Schmeling had knocked out Louis. The Fuehrer had crowed like the cock of the world's walk. Now it was time for the Brown Bomber to redeem himself and expose Hitler's lie of racial superiority.

My father came home from work that night excitedly waving the *New York Daily News* in my face. "You tell me all about the big fight!" he signed, his fists punching the air. "Joe Louis is fighting Max Schmeling. Joe has *my* name." He pointed to his chest. "Louis," he finger-spelled proudly.

My father was so excited about the fight that he rushed us

through the dinner my mother had spent hours preparing. Normally my father was always after me to eat more slowly, to chew each mouthful of food at least three times before swallowing—five times if it was calf's liver, which was exceedingly tough (and a dish I thoroughly detested). That night, however, after gulping his own food rather than chewing it, my father pushed his chair away from the table and signed to me, "*Let's go!*"

Twirling the dial, I soon tuned in to the broadcast of the fight. We were early. The prefight commentary by the announcer detailed the career of Joe Louis; that of Schmeling; the replay of their last fight; and the political significance of this rematch. The complexity of all this information surpassed by far both my understanding of current events and my signing sophistication. My father didn't care. All he was interested in was the fight itself.

Through the cloth speaker of my radio, I heard the bell ring. The crowd roared like a herd of wild beasts, the sound loud enough to wake the dead. My father just sat there, cocooned in serene silence, eyes locked on my hands, my face, and the radio, waiting for my hands to transform the invisible, unheard sound into the visible, understood sign.

The fight was on. The noise of the crowd, and the screaming voice of the announcer, poured in a torrent from my radio.

I struggled to sign what was happening, what I was hearing; struggled to keep up. But there were just too many raw sounds coming at me, all crowded together. Besides which, my signing vocabulary did not include signs for the boxing game. Oh, sure, I could sign *chicken*. That was easy, as the sign looked like a chicken. I could sign *corn*. (I was great with vegetables, as my father had taught me a garden of signs, a veritable farm full of signs.) But how to sign, *The Brown Bomber lands with an uppercut. Now he's jabbing Schmeling. Jab, jab, jab. There's no letup. Schmeling's eye is closing. Jab, jab, another jab to the eye. Joe Louis is killing him. Another uppercut. One* to the breadbasket. *Schmeling doubles over. OOOHH, that one will bring up his lunch.*

Pained frustration pinched my father's face as he looked un-comprehendingly at my incomprehensible, stuttering signs.

Equally frustrated, I leaped instinctively to my feet, swinging my arms, my childish fists extended. As I listened to each detail describing the action in the ring, I danced in circles in front of my father. I swung. I ducked. I bobbed. I weaved.

The punches I threw jolted my arms. The invisible impact of their landing shot up into my shoulders. I hunched in pain. But my face was Joe Louis's stoic mask, the one my father had shown me in the newspaper. I was killing Schmeling, that Nazi rat. Take *that!* How about *this!* Smack—my leather glove beat a tattoo on Schmeling's bloody puss. I was making hamburger out of his Aryan face, turning his Nazi body into mincemeat. So much for the Master Race.

I rose up on my toes and pursued the retreating, cowering Schmeling around the ring.

I heard the announcer scream, *He can run, but he can't hide. Louis has Schmeling on the ropes. He's pounding the bejesus out of him. HE'S DOWN! HE'S DOWN! SCHMELING'S DOWN! He's on the canvas.*

I dropped to the floor and lay spread-eagled on the rag rug.

Louis is standing over Schmeling.

I jumped up. I stared down at the rug impassively.

Schmeling's twitching.

I dropped to the floor. Rolled on my back. I twitched.

Schmeling's as still as a stone.

I was as still as a stone.

The referee waves Louis to a neutral corner.

I jumped up and followed his command, taking myself to what I deemed the neutral corner of the room.

ONE.

I signed in exaggerated emphasis the number one... *TWO*...two...*THREE*...three...*SCHMELING'S TRYING TO GET UP*...I fell down. I tried to rise ... and continued signing... *FOUR*...four...*FIVE*...five...*SCHMELING FALLS BACK TO THE CANVAS*...I fell back on the rug...*SIX*...six...I signed the number from the floor...*SEVEN*...seven...*EIGHT*... eight...*NINE*...nine...*TEN*...I made a fist, thrust my thumb up, and wiggled my hand furiously...*TEN*.

IT"S ALL OVER! SCHMELING'S OUT! I was signing like a maniac.

THE BROWN BOMBER IS THE HEAVYWEIGHT CHAMPION OF THE W.O.R.L.D.!

The noise from my radio was deafening.

I paraded around the room, arms upraised in victory; the tumultuous cheering pouring from the radio was music to my ears. "Take *that,* Adolf," I shouted at the top of my lungs.

My father was whooping and hollering and stamping his feet on the floor in wild unleashed joy.

The neighbors in the apartment below us were pounding on their ceiling with the end of a broom. Our next-door neighbors were banging on the wall between our apartments. The neighbors upstairs were stomping their feet on their floor. It was chaos.

My mother felt the noise from the floor below her feet, and the reverberations from the walls and ceiling, and ran into the room in alarm.

My deaf father heard nothing, but the look on his face said it all. He was laughing uproariously at my performance. Tears were coming out of his eyes and running down his cheeks.

"*Great fight!*" he signed, when he caught his breath, "*I understood everything!*"

I stood there in the middle of the ring, on the rag-rug canvas, exhausted but proud. Thank heavens, I thought, the fight had lasted less than one round. At my age I was in no shape to go the distance.

"I didn't know you knew how to box." He broke up again. "Your signing was great. Very clear." Then he laughed again; he couldn't contain himself.

Every year, after that performance, I was called upon to do it all over again, as Joe Louis fought his way through, and disposed of, an endless string of hapless opponents. Fortunately for me, in 1939 Joe Louis KO'd John Henry Lewis in the first round. No pile-driving man was this John Henry. He was sent to the canvas with one punch from the Brown Bomber's lethal fist.

My father was delighted, as was every other American, white and black.

The next year I turned seven, and Louis KO'd the oddly named, I thought, Johnny Paychek, in the second round. What the poor fellow had to do to earn his *paycheck* that night at the hands (fists) of Louis, I couldn't imagine. Personally I wouldn't go in the ring with Joe Louis for all the tea in China, let alone a mere *paycheck*.

The fight had gone one round further than I had fought before. My stamina was improving, and my signing as well. But still my father preferred for me to do my *special* signing for each match.

In 1941 both my endurance and my *special* signing were put to the test. On a warm, clear June evening, Joe Louis fought the upstart, much lighter and smaller but dangerous boxer, Billy Conn. My father was wild about this fight but terribly conflicted. He explained, as a runup to the bout, that Billy Conn was a Jew fighting for the heavyweight championship of the world. My father's head was with his religious brother, Conn, but his heart was with his long-time hero, Louis.

In anticipation of the fight, I went into training. My father had told me this would not be a one-round affair. Conn was too agile for that. He would stay out of reach of Louis's gloves. Therefore I needed to build up my wind. This time I might be called upon to go the distance. My father had signed to me that Conn could *dance*: the two fingers of his right hand formed a V, and the legs of the V *danced* across his open left hand. I could *see* Billy Conn's plan; he intended to *dance* his way to a decision. So I practiced dancing. When there was music on my radio, I had often seen my father dancing with my mother to the rhythms they both felt rising from the floorboards. With that image in my mind, I practiced.

By the night of the fight, I was ready; and now I had added my mother to the audience. She knew absolutely nothing about boxing and cared even less, but she seemed fascinated by my strange manic antics. Where my father laughed, she stared in utter amazement.

As they sat in obvious anticipation, I turned on my radio, and the fight began. I immediately went into a crouch and retreated, dancing. I was Billy Conn.

I ducked, I bobbed, I weaved around the room. Then I reversed position—now I was Joe Louis. I stalked, I threw ineffectual jabs in the air, into the space Conn had just vacated.

BONG! The end of round one.

And so it went, round after round. I retreated. I advanced. I ducked. I swung. And I danced. Boy, oh, boy, did I ever dance that night; I danced my eight-year-old heart out. The look of pure amazement and wonder on my mother's face was my reward.

Rounds ten, eleven, and twelve came and went, with the same result: Louis advancing, Conn dancing.

Billy Conn's on the balls of his feet, the announcer screamed. *He's dancing up a storm. Dancing. Dancing. Louis CAN'T CATCH HIM!*

Between rounds I sat in my *corner* (on the kitchen stool I had put there for that purpose). I was exhausted. How long, I wondered, could I—I mean, Billy Conn—last?

In the thirteenth round I had my answer. NOT LONG! *Conn is retreating. Conn is dancing, dancing . . . OOOPS, Louis has Conn trapped in the far corner of the ring. Conn looks desperate! He can't go left. He can't go right.* I stepped to my left. I stepped to my right. I was right back where I started from, trapped in the corner of the room.

Louis is shooting short punches to Conn's body. Conn is covering. Now Louis is punching to the head. Look at those punches! They only travel six inches, but what damage they're causing! I covered my head. My head bounced backward, then sideways. *Louis is a punching machine.* Then I reversed position and punched, punched, punched the air. I was Joe Louis, the Brown Bomber. I was a piston, a pile-driving man.

A tremendous roar shot out from the radio. *Conn's down. He's down! HE'S DOWN! Louis caught him right on the end of the jaw, between a bob and a weave.* My bobbing stopped. My weaving ended. My chin jerked up. *Conn's not dancing now.* I stopped dancing. I fell. *You can run, but you can't hide. Not from the Brown Bomber.* Lying on the rag rug of the *ring*, I knew that. "You can run, but you can't hide from Joe Louis."

The count droned its way to the inevitable conclusion of every one of Joe Louis's fights: *TEN! AND YOU'RE OUT!*

I leaped to my feet. I signed the inevitable numbers. I signed, *FINISHED!*

Wonderful! Wonderful! my father signed with obvious glee.

My mother just looked at me, as if seeing me for the first time, dumbstruck. She had never, in all the eight years of my life, witnessed such a signing performance. She was impressed.

In 1942 Joe Louis was inducted into the United States Army, along with a million other young boys and grown men. So were two of my mother's younger brothers: Harry, the quiet one, who, to the consternation of his mother, Celia, dated only Italian girls and was as chary of his words as he was of his money; and Milton, the youngest, who always had much to say, all of it directed at the failures of the capitalist system. In those simple days you volunteered; you did not wait to be drafted. It was a different war, a much different time.

There would be no more fights for the duration. Even kids knew what the "duration" meant—until the war was over. While this life-and-death struggle was being fought, everything in our young lives would be suspended for the "duration." And the cry went up all over Brooklyn, from a million mothers' lips, every time we asked for something: "Don't you know there's a war on!" That effectively ended every discussion.

The fact that I could now take a break from my *special* signing was okay with me, as I didn't think I had another round in me after that epic fight.

By 1946, however, when the war was over and Joe Louis resumed his boxing career, I was thirteen and stronger. Although my signing was now much more sophisticated and complex, my father insisted I continue to sign the fights as I had in the old days, with my *special* signing. So it was lucky for me that I had gained in strength and endurance, because Louis was now older and slower; he did not finish off his opponents as quickly as he once had. His bouts lasted many rounds. In 1947 he took the full fifteen rounds to gain a decision over the up-and-coming Jersey Joe Walcott. My father told me that that was my best performance as a fighter . . . he meant, signer.

In 1949 my father bought a DuMont television set. It had been reduced to $999. In those days the minimum wage was forty cents an hour. How my father managed this purchase is still beyond me. Being deaf, however, he viewed television not as a luxury but as a necessity.

With a plastic magnifying lens hooked to the front of the set by two wires, the eye-squinting eight-by-ten-inch screen was blown up to a highly distorted twenty-inch one. The resulting watery, convex image made us feel like goldfish looking out through the glass sides of a fish tank.

From now on my father would watch the fights on TV. There was no longer any need for me to sign them for him.

And so I retired, undefeated. In an extended ceremony, as my mother looked on with great amusement, my father crowned me with a newspaper hat that he had made out of a page from the day's paper; I was now the reigning world champion of boxing signs.

At the conclusion of the ceremony, my father signed to me wistfully, "Sure, I like to see the fights on TV now, but somehow they just don't have the same *excitement* as when you were in your prime." I felt good knowing this. But then he added, a gleam in his eye, a smile on his lips, "And they sure aren't nearly as funny."

Memorabilia

Sounds in the Night

One night, long after I had gone to bed, I was awakened by strange sounds in our otherwise silent apartment. It sounded as if someone were being beaten, the blows accompanied by grunts and muffled screams.

I jumped out of bed and rushed to my parents' bedroom.

Their door was closed, but it was never locked as, being deaf, they dared not shut out their hearing son.

I threw open the door, realizing as I did that this was where the sounds were coming from. Rushing into the dimly lighted room, I saw my father on top of my mother. He was grunting, and she was moaning. It was a frightening sight. I leaped on my father's bare back, screaming into his deaf ears, "Stop! Stop! You're killing my mother!"

In shocked reaction, my father bucked me off his back, and I landed with a thud on the wooden floor. On went the lights, and *bang bang bang* went the broom handle Mrs. Abromovitz thumped against the ceiling of her bedroom one floor below.

My father picked me up in his arms. I was crying. He stilled my shaking and gently wiped away my tears with the tips of his fingers.

"What's wrong?" he signed.

"Why are you beating my mother?" I signed. There are no fewer than five signs for *beat,* and I used every one of them.

My father watched my agitated performance in wonder, and upon its completion, he laughed uproariously.

Catching his breath, he signed, "Not *killing.*" Then after some thought he added, "We're *exercising.*" And with that he laughed some more.

I, of course, had no idea what was so funny. But I was reassured by his easy laughter that everything was all right.

This must have been true, as all throughout my childhood I heard my father and my mother exercising on a regular basis.

4

Another Child

$\mathcal{M}$y brother, Irwin, was born the year I turned four. My mother's parents, Celia and Max, had been against their deaf daughter having another child. Since they did not know with certainty why it was that she, their oldest child, had become deaf, they thought her children would most likely be deaf as well. The fact that I, their daughter's firstborn child, could hear was for them no less than a miracle. But, they reasoned, why take a chance on another miracle? Better to be safe than sorry. "No more children," her mother told her. "*One is enough!*" her father insisted, jabbing his forefinger at her.

My father agreed with both of them. This was rare—actually, unheard-of. My father considered his wife's parents to be little better than uneducated illiterate immigrants, barely off the boat. He was particularly incensed, though he never openly showed it, when they butted into his family's affairs. "Where do these immigrants get off telling me what to do?" his hands would mutter. "Just because I'm deaf they think me stupid; nothing more than a child." But as my father worshiped his beautiful wife, who in turn had always basked in the undiluted love of her mother, he held his tongue—hands actually. In moments of extreme agitation, such as when his wife's sister, Mary, wrote out his father-in-law's dire warnings about how innocent and childlike and irresponsible my father was because he was a "deaf and dumb mute," my father would literally sit on his hands so as to contain them, as if they possessed an independent will to strangle this Hungarian Gypsy fool.

But on this point, that one child was enough, he found himself in agreement with his in-laws. As was always the case, my mother ignored her family's wishes entirely. She dearly loved her mother, Celia, but had always known, with a certainty beyond her years, that she was different from her mother and the rest of her hearing family. Her life now was with her own family, her deaf family. And she was determined to talk her husband into a second child.

She had been arguing with him about this for over three years—ever since they both concluded that my hearing was in no danger of being lost. He pointed out to her that they could much better afford to provide for one child than for two. It was 1937, and the Depression still gripped the country. "What if the newspaper cuts back my hours?" he argued intelligently. "I want another little baby," my mother signed sweetly. "What if I have to go back on the lobster shift? How will you manage at night?" he pointed out reasonably. "Myron will help me," my mother said.

All argument was useless; my mother wanted another baby in the house. And as my father adored my mother, he gave in. The outcome of this issue, as with all others, was never in doubt; what Sarah wanted, Sarah would have. And so she and Lou had another child.

My brother, Irwin, was born hearing. (Actually, ninety percent of all children born to deaf parents can hear.) When it was announced, at the hospital, that the new baby could hear, both sides of the family assumed that the *curse* of deafness had been broken.

And with this baby, neither my mother's nor my father's family felt the need to make regularly scheduled weekend visits to our apartment for the yearlong ritual of banging on pots and pans.

*F*rom the day my mother came home from the hospital, I was required to be my brother's surrogate parent. No longer did my mother have to rely, as she had with me, on a ribbon tied from her arm to her new baby's foot. That velvet ribbon was now replaced by me. For my mother, I was a much more satisfactory connection between her newborn son and herself. After all, a ribbon can't speak in sign.

My brother's crib was placed alongside my bed. When he awoke at night, crying for his bottle, it was my job to wake my mother. When he awoke at night with a stomachache, it was my job to wake my mother. When he awoke at night, fussy and fretful, it was my job to wake my mother. But as he grew older, he would sometimes awaken simply because he was no longer sleepy; then I would play with him as he lay on his back in his crib.

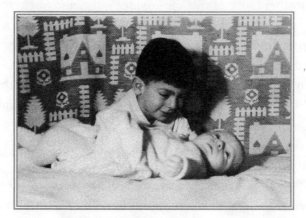

Irwin and I

Irwin was an extremely placid baby, somewhat on the chubby side, quick to make eye contact and just as quick to smile and giggle. When I looked at him, he would often cycle his legs and wave his arms in what appeared to me to be great excitement. I, in turn, would wave my arms back at him to see if I could get an even greater response. And if this failed, I would make faces at him. Having unconsciously learned from my parents the exaggerated facial expressions that are a part of deaf grammar, I would raise my eyebrows high and fatten my cheeks to bursting, to see if he would imitate me.

It was at such times—in the middle of the night—that I thought to teach my brother to speak. Our house was a silent one, and other than the voices that emanated from my radio, I heard no speech. But if my brother could learn to speak, I reasoned, I would have a companion, one whom I could talk to and who, in turn, would talk back to me. I was curious as to what his speaking voice would sound like. Being the child of deaf parents, I was acutely aware of the sound of speech—the way the people on my block articulated words, their accents, and in the case of my friend Jerry's immigrant Italian father, the music of their speech. And so as my brother looked up at me—wide awake, and not in the least bit sleepy—I would look down at him and repeat words over and over again, hoping to elicit a response. Of course, at that early age none was forthcoming. Nonetheless I was determined to be for my baby brother the human replacement for the radio that had spoken to me when I was a baby. And in time, at an unusually early age, he did begin to speak.

A black-and-white picture of my brother at about the age of three hangs on my wall of family photographs. An extraordinarily cute child, he is towheaded, with a hank of fluffy hair hanging down over his left eye. His look is one of pure Huck Finn mischief. His face is round, with cheeks so plump he might be hiding a small knobby crabapple in each one—to tease my mother, no doubt. His eyes are the outstanding feature of his face; they are large, dark, and lively. A deep shining intelligence illuminates them; they are looking off to the side, completely unaware of the camera, as if planning the next prank. The satisfied smile that forms on his lips suggests his sense of anticipation.

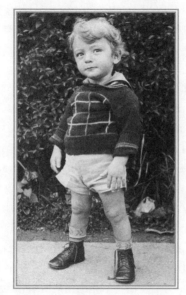

Irwin, circa 1940

My brother is wearing a sweater knitted for him by our mother. It bunches up around his waist, and the sleeves are rolled back to the middle of his arms. His chubby hands hang straight down, fat fingers like ten little sausages pointing to the ground. My mother was a skilled and inventive knitter and seamstress (no need, ever, for *patterns*), but she always made every garment too large. "So you won't outgrow it," she always signed, when I would complain about some article of clothing she had made for me that hung halfway to the floor. (Come to think of it, in all the years I was a child I never seemed to outgrow a single thing she made for me.)

Beneath the hand-knit sweater my brother wears a rumpled pair of shorts. The shorts expose his bare legs, which are also pudgy, with a pair of dimples at each knee. Hand-knitted patterned socks peek above his high-top laced leather shoes. One bow has become untied, and the laces trail on the ground at his foot. This photograph of my brother, taken by our father with his Brownie box camera, could have been painted by Gainsborough.

Two years later my brother would have his first epileptic seizure.

One night I was awakened by sounds I had never heard before. I groped for the switch on my bedside lamp, and when I turned the knob, I saw a sight that made me gasp. In the bed next to mine, the location he had slept in all of his life, my brother was gripped with an epileptic grand mal seizure. His eyes were rolled back in his head, only the whites showing. The skin on his face was drawn tightly to his skull. His mouth was clamped shut, with the edge of his tongue protruding, and blood was spurting all over his white pillowcase. His body was as rigid as a wooden plank. He squirmed and writhed and jerked about. His arms and legs flew in every direction, like the demented arms of a windmill. Sweat was flying from his body. I was stunned, turned to stone.

I couldn't say afterward if his seizure had lasted one minute or an hour. Time had no meaning. My entire focus of attention was on my brother as he was transformed into a creature beyond my comprehension.

When he was finally still—which happened, it seemed, in an instant—he lay there drenched in sweat, his face covered in blood, completely unconscious.

In time—I can't say how long—I went to get my father and mother. When I jerked my father awake, the look on my face threw him into a panic, and my mother screamed. Rushing into my bedroom, they saw a sight that is the stuff of every parent's nightmare: their son covered in blood, blood everywhere on his sheets and pillow, while he lay, scarcely breathing, as if dead.

While my mother held his now limp, boneless, virtually lifeless body in her arms, my father tenderly wiped the blood from his body and face with a damp cloth, searching for its source.

That evening was the beginning of a year of nonstop, nightly seizures. Every night when it was time to go to sleep, my father tied a cloth strip from my arm to my brother's arm as he lay in his bed, which was now drawn right alongside my own. On my bedside table was a selection of wooden tongue depressors, which my father had wrapped thickly in gauze. My instructions were simple. "When you feel the cloth jerk, that's the signal that Irwin will be going into a seizure. Get up immediately. Straddle your brother, force his jaws open, clear his tongue away from his teeth, and slip the tongue depressor between his jaws, making sure, doubly sure, that his tongue is clear of his teeth. Then, and only then, remove your fingers from his mouth. Be sure, but be quick. When he goes into convulsions, straddle his body between your thighs, and hold him as still as you can. Whatever you do, don't let him jerk himself off his bed." He added, "Your mother and I are counting on you. You can hear. We are deaf." I was nine years old.

I became quite adept at these esoteric skills. I slept lightly, never dreaming, and would snap awake the instant my brother stiffened, which happened each night that first year, as regularly as a clock alarm. His arm would jerk, the cloth stretched between us would yank on my arm, and I would leap onto his body, straddling him between my thighs. A gauze-wrapped tongue depressor found its way into my hand without any conscious thought on my part. Holding his mouth open, I thrust the depressor into his mouth and pushed aside his tongue. Most nights I was successful. Some nights I managed to get my fingers out of his mouth before it snapped shut, but I was not able to clear his tongue completely from his clenching jaws. Then the blood would fly. Occasionally I was not quick enough to remove my fingers before his jaws clamped shut, and then my blood would mingle with his.

Deep into that year my brother began to have episodes of repeated seizures. When this happened, I had to awaken our downstairs neighbor and ask to use her phone so that I could call 911 (or whatever its equivalent was sixty-five years ago). She did not once complain. When the ambulance arrived, I accompanied my father and my unconscious brother to Coney Island Hospital. There I went through the usual routine of being my father's ears and voice. But in this situation I was also the voice and ears of my unconscious brother.

I instinctively knew that my father hated being in this situation, helpless because of his deafness. And the unthinking, uncaring, unsympathetic treatment he received from the hospital staff—all of them, from ambulance driver to orderly to nurse and doctor— was deeply painful to him. Not one of them had a moment for my father. I, on the other hand, was the center of their attention. As an adult with children of my own, I can very well imagine the humiliation my father must have felt at those times: ignored and dismissed as if he were a child of no consequence, while I was spoken to almost as the parent of my little brother.

My brother's epileptic seizures were to last for five years, gradually diminishing in frequency. During that time he drank a daily concoction of powerful sedatives—including phenobarbital— which transformed him into a virtual zombie. And although he entered school at the appropriate age, he never seemed to be fully aware of what was going on in his classes; he always seemed to be sleepwalking. As he told me many years later about his school years, "I just didn't get it." How could he, drugged into oblivion by sedatives that would never be prescribed for an epileptic child today?

Eventually my brother's seizures ceased. But by then my mother's heart was broken.

My own feelings toward my brother were complex. From the age of nine, my age at the time my brother's seizures began, until I discovered the escape that high school football afforded me, my love for my brother was infused with resentment for his ceaseless need of me. He was never merely my younger brother—that could never be, because of the sticky web of responsibility in which I was forever entangled. Almost from the moment he was born I was responsible for "minding" him. That meant that my primary focus was on him and not on me; on his needs, not mine. Needs that in my mother's and father's eyes, of necessity, took precedence over mine. With the onset of his epileptic seizures, my needs were not merely overlooked—they were obliterated.

And, of course, my brother was my complete responsibility at night.

As he grew older, I was tasked not only with teaching him how to speak but acting as translator between him and our parents. In time he acquired a basic proficiency in sign language from casual instructions from our parents. But for much of our childhood, the more complex flow of language between them and him was through me.

My first language had been sign. Because of me, my brother's first language would be spoken. When he was a baby, I thought it would be fun to get him to speak. But soon it became work. During his acquisition of spoken language, it was my responsibility to keep my parents abreast of his progress. After all, being deaf, how could they possibly know if my tutelage was succeeding?

I loved my brother and felt deeply sorry for him, but I experienced his dependence on me, and his unvoiced expectation that I would fulfill the role of caretaker, as a burden. And while I adored my father, he, too, was a burden on me, one that I often wished I did not have to shoulder.

Why was I the only kid on my block, certainly in all of Brooklyn, probably in the entire world, who was responsible for an epileptic brother and two deaf parents? I wondered, bathed in the warm waters of self-pity. *Why couldn't I be like everyone else on my block? It just wasn't fair,* I thought. *I'm just a kid.*

I had found within myself a state of dull resignation at being the son of deaf parents, with all the obligations that entailed. But my epileptic brother, and the added responsibility that he created for me, was another matter. It was one thing to be singled out on my street as the son of the "deafies" in 3A, which is all my parents were ever known as on our block. Not as Louis and Sarah; not as Mr. and Mrs. Uhlberg; but rather as the "deaf and dumb mutes in 3A." This unthinking consignment as objects of curiosity, and even pity, was something I had adapted to. But to be minding my brother in the street on a sunny afternoon when my father was at work and my mother was busy cleaning our apartment, and have him suddenly, inexplicably, stiffen, go glassy-eyed, and fall as a dead man to the pavement, was another thing entirely. Lying there, helpless, he would spasm into convulsions, his body as rigid as if petrified, transformed in an instant from an organic being into a stony replica of a little boy.

My friends would swarm around us, staring slack-jawed at the sight of my brother thrashing around uncontrollably on the sidewalk, often sliding off the curb and into the gutter. All the while I was astride him, as if riding a bucking horse.

Through some compensatory sense of telepathy granted to the deaf by an uncaring god with a perverse sense of humor, my mother would often sense the event and would hang from our third-floor bedroom window, keening in her deaf voice at the sight.

*T*here were times when I would come into our apartment, after playing all afternoon on our block, and catch my father and mother deep in conversation. When they were that engrossed with each other's signs, they were completely oblivious to my presence. If I wanted their attention, I would have to stomp my feet repeatedly on our wooden floor (and risk the downstairs neighbor banging a broom on her ceiling) or position myself between their flying hands. But once when I came home, I was so astonished by what my father was saying to my mother that I could only watch.

"Why didn't you *listen* to me, Sarah? I told you, one child was enough. Now look, we have a poor boy who has fits all night and who sleeps all day. And when he does wake up, he's never fully awake, what with all the medication he takes. I told you, but you wouldn't listen."

"Why do you tell me this now?" my mother signed. "What's done is done. There's no going back. I took the hot baths you asked me to, every night for a month. They didn't work, and I'm glad they didn't. It was God's will that he be born. It's not his fault he's sick like this. We'll manage. *Leave me alone!*"

"Don't talk to me about God. What did God ever do for me?" my father's hand jerked up above his head and dropped, as he signed "the One above." My father's sign for God was abrupt, dismissive. "He made me deaf and spared my sisters and brother. And he made you deaf as well, while sparing *your* brothers and sister."

I could not stand to see my father and mother arguing like this. It was rare, and in some deep way it scared me, as if I had become unmoored, adrift between my deaf parents and my sick brother. I ran outdoors, seeking escape in the company of my friends, and did not return until I heard my mother calling for me from our apartment window. Then I came back, and they were no longer arguing about my brother, or my father's indifferent God.

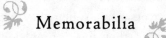

Memorabilia

Trains, Trains, Trains

The day I turned seven my father came home from work carrying a large gaily wrapped box under his arm. It was a train set.

"This train," his hands informed me, "is the Blue Comet!" Sitting on the floor, he assembled the tracks. Carefully he set the locomotive with its coal car and passenger cars on the track.

"The Blue Comet," my father's fingers spelled the name with exquisite care, "is ready to roll."

At bedtime he took the tracks apart and put the train back in the box.

The next night he came home with yet another big box under his arm.

"This train," he announced, finger-spelling the name, "is the Pennsylvania Flyer."

Adding new sections of track to the old, he positioned the new train with its boxcars and caboose behind the Blue

Comet. Placing an engineer's cap on his head, he said, "Let 'er roll!"

It took quite some time that night to disassemble the tracks and store the trains under my bed.

The next day my father came home with another large box under his arm. He put on striped-gray engineer's overalls and adjusted his engineer's cap.

Sitting on the floor, he signed, "ALL ABOARD!" and sent the Blue Comet, the Pennsylvania Flyer, and the new Allegheny Express rushing after one another, *clickety-clack, clickety-clack,* down the tracks curled around my bedroom floor.

On Saturday my father brought home large panels of plywood and assorted packages in all shapes and sizes. He put his big saw and all his tools in my bedroom, closing the door behind him. On the door he had hung a Do Not Disturb sign. "This means YOU," he boldly wrote across the sign. "Son Myron," he added at the bottom, for perfect clarity.

That night he stood with me at my closed bedroom door.

"Close your eyes," his hands commanded.

I did, and seconds later when he told me to open them again, I saw that my bedroom was now filled with a huge table. To make room, my father had pushed both my bed and my brother's bed against the far wall. On the table there were train tracks going every which way, up and down, in and out, over and under, twisting and curving. Waiting on the track sat three locomotives, blue, red, and black. Coal cars, tenders, passenger cars, freight cars, flatcars, and three cabooses. A lone Heinz Pickle boxcar trailed behind them.

There were tunnels, bridges, houses, and stations. There were grass-covered hills over which miniature cows and a flock of tiny white sheep grazed. Between the hills rushed rivers and streams made of glass, telephone poles fashioned from pencils, and fences made of toothpicks. Toy cars sat in arrested motion on blacktopped roads lined with perfect little streetlamps.

And everywhere I looked there were little people, frozen in midmotion. My father was good with his hands. He spoke with his hands in more ways than one.

As I stood there by his side, gazing in astonished wonder at the scene spread out before me, he turned off the ceiling light and went to the control panel he had built into the exact center of the table. Suddenly the table burst into light. Every tiny bulb behind every wax-paper window in every miniature house blazed on; all the perfect little streetlamps sprinkled perfect specks of light on the black road below; the signals at track crossings began to insistently blink yellow, then red; bridges wore necklaces trimmed in light, and the train sheds, no longer dark, displayed their illuminated cardboard nooks and crannies.

As I stared, my hands forgotten at my sides, unable to sign a single word, my father put the engineer's cap on my head, signing, "You take over, chief. Happy birthday!"

I don't think I slept a wink that night. And I never for a moment thought of taking off my engineer's cap.

When my brother turned four, among his many presents was a smaller version of my engineer's hat. Up until then I had strictly forbidden him to touch the control panel. "Look. DON'T TOUCH!" was my constant admonition. But now that he had his own engineer's cap, I magnanimously allowed him to control the magnetic derrick that offloaded the freight cars. I soon regretted this gesture, as from then on he insisted I stop the trains every time they passed the derrick.

As I grew older, I lost interest in my trains, and my brother took over. It thrilled him to run the three sets of trains simultaneously at excessive speeds, until they jumped the track—much to my father's consternation.

Eventually Irwin also lost interest in the train set. And one day my father dismantled the whole project and sent it off to a younger cousin of ours—along with my engineer's hat.

5

Heaven

*A*lthough I could not help but resent my brother's dependence on me, I was also ashamed of my feelings. I knew guilt at an age when most children have no sense of such an emotion. When this toxic brew would overcome me, I often sought to escape to the one place where I could be truly alone—the roof of our apartment building.

The roof was my personal heaven, my sanctuary. On a summer's day I would sit in solitary silence, my back to the low warm brick wall that edged the roof, with nothing but blue sky above my head. On that roof, on such a day, my ears were not filled with the incessant sounds of my Brooklyn block; nor were my eyes filled to overflowing with the incessant signs of my father, or the image of my brother suddenly stiffening and dropping to the ground.

On the roof I would read every copy of my extensive comic book collection, over and over again. I would get lost in the adventures recounted in these stories—the close calls, the speeding trains, the angry lions, the nefarious crooks—and dream I was a normal kid.

* * *

𝒯he roof wasn't just my own, of course; it was communal property. On summer evenings the neighbors would gather there to cool off, sitting in family groups on blankets spread over the graveled tarpaper, covered edge to edge with cold chicken, beer, lemonade, potato salad, cakes, and cookies. We kids would migrate from blanket to blanket, begging a cookie or a drumstick, for no other reason than to see if somebody else's food tasted any different from our mother's efforts.

Tuesday nights in summer were special. As the sky darkened over Coney Island, fireworks were shot up into the sky over the Atlantic, where they burst into incandescent blooms of light against the purpled horizon. On rooftops all over Bensonhurst, collective *OOOHHHHs* and *AAAHHHHs* rose to the heavens, in a chorus of appreciation. For once my father's deaf voice blended into the rest and was unremarked upon. And my little brother sat mercifully still, watching with open mouth and glazed eyes, nodding in time with the exploding of each new pyrotechnic display.

𝒪n one side of the roof was Frankie's pigeon coop. Behind the chicken wire, sitting shoulder to shoulder on doweled roosts, were hundreds of gray pigeons, all facing in the same direction.

I would hide behind the brick chimney when I heard Frankie open the heavy metal roof door. And from there, unseen, I would watch him talk to his pigeons for hours. Frankie was not dumb, but he talked baby talk to those birds. They seemed to like it, so who was I to object? Besides, I knew sign language, not pigeon language. Maybe Frankie's words were making sense to the birds. They sure seemed to be listening.

After a while he opened the cage door, and with a long bamboo pole he shooed the birds off their roost and into the air. They flew as one, like a gray cloud, up, up into the blue sky over our roof, shedding a mist of slowly falling feathers in their wake, leaving their white calling cards on the black macadam below.

With the bamboo pole Frankie waved the flock into ever-expanding circles, extending over Avenue P and Kings Highway.

Not content with that feat of magic, he waved the pole ever more vigorously, until the pigeons wheeled out of sight.

The first time I ever watched this happen, I thought, the big show-off, now he's lost his pigeons. Now who will he have to talk his baby talk to? *Not me!* Just as I thought those pigeons must surely be flying over the George Washington Bridge to New Jersey, and from there to California, Frankie stamped the end of his pole on the roof, and miraculously they reappeared in the Brooklyn sky. In ever-diminishing circles they returned to our roof, where in a graceful fall, single file, they reentered the coop.

Frankie closed the cage door and told them in his pigeon language that they were beautiful. They sat, pigeon feet clinging to their perch, bobbing their heads in total agreement.

When the weather was clear, I would go to my roof with my official enemy plane-spotter cards and my father's binoculars. Kneeling behind the brick outer wall, so as not to be seen by the enemy pilots, I would look out over Coney Island. That's the direction the German planes would come from. Why they would come to Brooklyn was a question that never entered my mind. Perhaps to bomb Nathan's Famous, whose food sustained the morale of every citizen of Brooklyn. The loss of their franks and buttered corn would be a near-mortal blow.

Those German planes never came. They must have known from enemy intelligence that I was on guard, ever vigilant, protecting Brooklyn.

* * *

*M*y roof was not just a summer place.

In the winter, after a heavy snowfall, when the rest of the kids ran down into the street, I would go in the other direction. Pushing the roof door open against the piled-up snow was a challenge. But once accomplished, I had the roof all to myself. I would spend hours trekking through the accumulation of snow, my footprints the only ones disturbing its smooth surface.

When enough snow had fallen, I made enormous snowballs. They were cannonball size. Then bomb size. These I proceeded to lob over the wall onto the unsuspecting neighbors below. I was not the bombardier of a B-17 Flying Fortress, and I had no Norden bombsight, but my accuracy was positively uncanny.

6

Clothes Make the Boy

*O*ne morning toward the end of summer, my father shook me awake with his strong printer's hands. An annual tradition was about to be set in motion.

"School starts thirty days from now," his hands fairly screamed at me. "There is a big sale on boys' suits at Mr. R. and H. Macy's store today. We must hurry!"

My father, who had never owned a single suit as a boy, now insisted that his son have a new one every year. Every summer, about a month before the beginning of the school year, as regular as clockwork, the ritual of buying a new suit for me would begin. And once begun, the ritual was my signal that summer was over. Oh, sure, the calendar on my wall still said "August," but this day signaled that the calendar was lying; I could almost feel the chill of autumn on my bare skin.

"Time is short. Hurry! Hurry!" he signed with an insistent choppy movement of his hands. "We've got to get a move on before all the good stuff is snapped up."

"Good stuff? Snapped up?" I mumbled under my breath. I

didn't have to mumble. My father wouldn't hear me. He was deaf. But I did have to be careful, because he could read my lips.

Slowly I dragged myself out of bed. I was in no rush to begin this day. A day that would bring me no joy. A day that was sure to be wall-to-wall embarrassment as I played the go-between, negotiating the transaction of buying a suit with my father on one side, and a bunch of unsympathetic, impatient, hearing salesmen all working on commission on the other side. For them, time was money. My father had all the time in the world to select just the right suit for his son. They had none to spare.

"We'll start with Mr. Bloomingdale," my father's hands informed me. "His basement has a ton of suits. All with two pants. And he has the best prices in the city."

Best prices? I thought. Sure, but in all the time we shopped there, we never bought a single suit. Bloomingdale's basement was just that, the starting point in an endless day.

"Who knows?" my father added. "If we're lucky, we'll find a two-for-one sale."

At the end of two subway rides that took us from the far reaches of the oceanside fringe of Brooklyn to the treeless streets of Manhattan, we exited the station into a world far different from the one we had left behind. Lexington Avenue and 59th Street on the island of Manhattan was to West Ninth Street at the outer edge of Brooklyn "as different as St. Petersburg was to Odessa," my grandmother Celia always said. That is, when she said anything at all.

Holding my hand, my father marched me across Lexington Avenue, already clogged with trucks and cabs manned by sweating and swearing drivers, their bleating horns and curses falling unheard on my father's deaf ears. Safely arriving on the other side of the avenue, my father dropped my hand, and now, freed from my grasp, his hands flung excitement in every direction. "What a great day this is! Me with my son Myron, out to buy a suit. A *beautiful* day. Listen! Can you hear the sunshine sound on the ladies' red dress in the window? And look at the light of the sunshine! See how it breaks up into diamonds in the puddle at the curb! Smell the exhaust from the automobiles! Can you taste it on the back of your tongue?"

For my father, who could not hear, every other sense was heightened to compensate for his loss. He even claimed to "hear" the sound of color.

Leaving the sunlit street, we descended into the artificial light of Bloomingdale's basement. That's where the two-for-one suits were located. And there were thousands of them hanging in that vast, poorly lit room. I could swear my father licked his lips in anticipation at the sight of all that wool.

Being ever practical by nature, he always began by instructing me to try on the suits that were sewn of the heaviest wool fabrics. Pattern didn't matter: plaids, stripes, herringbone. Weave was not an issue: serge, gabardine, worsted. Price was of no concern. Nothing mattered except sheer weight.

"These are great," his hands assured me, while his mobile face accompanied his happy hands with a big self-satisfied smile. "These are bulletproof suits."

"Great," my doubting hands said. "These suits would serve me well in the invasion of Europe. What German soldier would shoot at a kid from Brooklyn wearing a plaid suit like this? And if he did, how surprised he'd be when the bullets bounced off the lapels."

I could tell by my father's expression that my jokes fell flat. They did not deter him at all. His only response was "Follow me."

Off to the dressing room we went, my father with ten wool suits clutched to his chest, me following dutifully behind. The way his arms drooped, I figured the suits must have weighed about a hundred pounds.

"Where is a salesman?" my father signed in the suddenly deserted room. "They're never around when you need one."

I didn't have the heart to tell my father that at the sight of us, every salesman in the place had scurried off, as the cockroaches did late at night when I turned on the light in our kitchen to get a glass of water. Our fruitless, sales-less annual visits had not been forgotten by those who worked on commission: no sale, no commission. Every summer in came my father, and off ran the salesmen.

"Never mind," my father signed. "I know Mr. Bloomingdale's inventory like I know the contents of my closet. It never changes."

Suit after suit I tried on. Modeling each one for my father while being rotated by him, like a chicken on a spit, I stood in front of a huge tilted floor mirror.

"Not right," he said. "Bunches up in the back. Makes you look like a little hunchback man. The same as in that sad movie. You know, the man who rings the church bell. Try this one next.

"Too tight. Try the next one.

"Plaid makes you look fat. Now you look like a little fat man-boy. Like Lou Costello." He laughed, but as my father looked not in the least like Bud Abbott, I did not join in his hilarity. Actually, by then I usually felt like crying.

"Try this one.

"The stripes make you look like a string bean boy. Green suit makes you look good enough to eat. Like a vegetable. Maybe we'll take you home and Mother Sarah will cook son Myron in his new green string bean suit."

Oh, what a day this would be! His jokes were as unfunny to me as mine had been to him.

"Try this one on next."

Suit after itchy wool suit I tried on and modeled for my father. None were satisfactory to his eye.

Hours passed. Suit after suit was plucked off the rack and brought to me in the dressing room. Suit after suit took its place on the dressing room wall, then the dressing room bench, and finally, stacked up neatly, on the dressing room floor.

When my father had exhausted every single suit in my size, as well as sizes I could never grow into before they went out of style—if they had ever been in style—he threw up his hands, announcing, "Well, that's it for Mr. Bloomingdale. He had his chance. We gave him first crack."

"But we never, *ever* buy a suit from Bloomingdale's," I pointed out to him. "We come here every year. I try on every suit they have in my size, even sizes too large for me. 'You'll grow into this someday,' you say. And after all those solids and plaids and stripes and herringbones, you always say, 'Well, that's it for Mr. Bloomingdale.'"

"Quality," he signed patiently, as if explaining to a backward child. "That's what we're after. Only the very best suit is good enough for my son Myron."

Holding my hand in his left hand while signing abbreviated signs with his right, my father launched us into the stream of traffic on Lexington Avenue.

"Next stop, Mr. R. and H. Macy. Largest store in the world." I looked at the expansiveness of my father's sign as he let go of me for a moment, his hands spread wide describing the size of R. H. Macy, and my heart dropped at the mere thought of the visit.

Safely on the other side of the avenue, after my father had stared down a fast-approaching taxi, daring it to hit us, we boarded a bus, then ducked into the subway for a short ride downtown.

Climbing out of the station at 34th Street, we stood at the entrance to the home of Mr. R. and H. Macy. An enormous place, it occupied an entire square block, street to street, avenue to avenue. I couldn't begin to imagine how many suits in my size it might contain. I wondered if Mr. R. and H. Macy was open twenty-four hours a day, seven days a week. There was no way we could get through all the suits in this place before school started.

With a look of fierce determination on his face, my father took my hand. We whirled into the store through the giant revolving door. Along with a score of other shoppers, we were swept into a waiting elevator, which rose with a sudden acceleration, before quickly dumping us into the middle of the suit department.

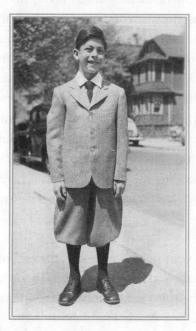

*In my new
R. & H. Macy suit*

Spread out before us was a vast ocean of suits, row upon endless row, quite possibly all the suits that had ever been made, except for those poor two-pants-per-jacket versions hanging in

Mr. Bloomingdale's emporium, which had utterly failed my father's quality test.

The thought of the sheer quantity of sheep that had been clipped to produce the wool that had been woven into the cloth that was used to make these endless flocks of suits staggered my imagination. In my mind's eye, I could see all those poor, cold, naked, shivering sheep huddled together on a grassy hill somewhere in Scotland, trying to stay warm.

I glanced up at my father and saw a look of pure happiness spread across his face, which soon gave way to a mask of determined yet optimistic resolve.

Taking a firm grip on my hand, he waded bravely into the oncoming waves of hanging suits, stretching out to the horizon of banked elevators, with me following haplessly in his wake.

Now the second act of this dreadful play began—and this would also be a long one, as Mr. R. and H. Macy had if possible even more suits than Mr. Bloomingdale, and even fewer salesmen in evidence, for the clothing salesmen in Macy's also saw my father coming and if anything ran faster than those at Bloomingdale's. Undaunted, as resolute as Richard Burton seeking the source of the Nile, my father trudged forward, leading me by the hand as if I were John Hanning Speke: *By God, we'll find the source of the Nile or die trying.*

*O*nce we had returned to our neighborhood at the end of one of these epic days, the annual purchase held securely in the hands of my triumphant father, the third act of our annual drama would begin. As we exited the Sea Beach line subway stop at Kings Highway, my father would sign, "You've been a good boy today. I'm proud of you. You were a big help to me. And you were fun company. Now for your reward."

Our neighborhood candy store was our Arabian Nights Bazaar, containing not just candy but other delights, some of them ordinary and practical, some exotic. Here we bought our brand-new spaldeens (when we had split the old one in two, with a perfectly executed swing of a sawed-off broomstick) and chocolate Kisses in their silver wrappers. Button candy, dripped as dots onto tissue-thin paper, was sold by the inch, each multicolored sugary button to be sucked singly into our greedy mouths and savored (when we weren't trying to extract the bits of paper stuck on the backs of the buttons from between our teeth). The most exciting purchase of all was the wax lips. Ruby red, perfectly molded, and shaped into a perpetual pouty smile in wax, they were as flavorful as a Yahrzeit candle. But with these bulbous red lips clenched firmly between our front teeth, we kids would parade gleefully around the neighborhood, pressing our faces into the thighs of every grown-up we encountered. The *why* of it all escapes me to this day.

"Choose anything you want," my father signed. "Even two things today."

Wow, I thought. *Where do I begin?*

My father was the model of patience. "Take your time," he said. And so in unconscious imitation of him in the department stores, I looked at every comic book in the candy store, handled every small toy, and fingered every small trinket except for that near-universal favorite, the tin clicking frog. Every kid in Brooklyn knew that by repeatedly clicking a clicking frog, they could drive their parents nuts in five minutes flat. But that didn't work with mine, of course. Finally I settled on a Batman comic and a set of wax lips. "I'll wear them when we get home," I told my father. "Mother won't recognize me." My father smiled at the image of me walking through our front door, smiling like an idiot at my mother with my ruby-red lips.

"Can we get a set for Irwin?" I asked my father. "That way Mother will be doubly surprised."

Readily agreeing, my father, like the great director he was, staged the conclusion of the final act: egg cream sodas for both of us. And so the curtain came down, the play was over: I had my new suit, and he had his day alone with his son.

7

A Day in the City

I had never gotten closer to where my father worked than the feeling of a newspaper hat on my head, which he made from the paper he brought home every evening. But one day when he was on vacation, he took me to the *New York Daily News* building.

That morning he selected the clothes I would wear—that year's new suit, of course. Then he dressed himself in his best clothes and freshly polished shoes. After kissing my mother and brother goodbye, we went down into the street. As dressed up as I had ever seen him, hat rakishly angled on his head, he took my hand in his, and we walked to the Kings Highway stop on the BMT subway, where we descended the stairs and stood on the platform for the train to Manhattan. As we waited for the train to arrive, I couldn't help but notice how happy my father seemed.

The train took us into the city, where we transferred to another train, which took us to a stop near my father's workplace.

Exiting the subway, my father took my hand and urged me to walk faster. Soon we arrived in front of the *New York Daily News* building.

I stood with my father outside the ornate, glass-covered entrance to the lobby. No matter how far backward I bent, I simply could not see the top of the building. Leaning back as far as my spine would allow, I struggled in vain to see the top of this snow-white tower. The rows of vertical white-brick panels rose from the city sidewalk, where I stood in my heavily shined shoes, straight up into a limitless blue sky, where they seemed to merge into a single point, thirty-seven floors above my head. Blimpy white clouds looked like fat dirigibles sailing slowly overhead, preparing to dock on the roof, just as real zeppelins once did on the roof of the Empire State Building.

Pushing our way through the revolving door, we entered the splendor of the high-domed lobby of the *New York Daily News*. I had never seen anything like it. The vast space was dark, lit in strategic spots by recessed lighting. The floor we stood on was of slick terrazzo squares. And there in front of me, sitting halfway down a wide deep hole, behind a chrome railing, revolved an enormous globe. The globe spun on its axis, basking in the rays shed by the soft spotlights positioned overhead; it was illuminated from below by the lights shining from a circle of glass steps that rose out of the depths to the brass belt around the equator.

It was a solitary, endlessly spinning object, bathed in light, in the otherwise dark lobby. My first sight of that magnificent spinning ball, which represented the earth where I lived, took my breath away. Every known country was outlined in bright colors. Every city, noted. The seven blue oceans divided the continents. The North Pole whitely capped the top of the revolving globe, while its distant relative, the South Pole, completed the picture deep down in the well. I was awestruck, although I later learned that the genius who had designed this magnificent spectacle had set the globe to turning in the wrong direction when it was initially installed.

As I stared in amazement, I began to wonder where my block was. And for that matter, where was *Brooklyn*? I then realized what a giant ball would be necessary to show West Ninth Street. It would have to be at least the size of the Wonder Wheel in Coney Island. And—my imagination was in full flight now—the lobby that housed such a globe would have to be the size of . . . what? I simply couldn't imagine. As for the size of the building that could house the lobby that contained a globe the size of the Wonder Wheel—I had reached the outer limit of what even my fervid imagination was capable of.

"Nice," I signed.

After I'd had my fill of the lobby, we rode the elevator, ascending in a stomach-dropping whoosh to the floor on which my father worked. The elevator car stopped with a suddenness that threatened to bring up my breakfast.

From the moment I left the quiet of the elevator car, and penetrated the wall of sound that greeted me when we arrived at the printing press floor, I literally could not hear myself think. The noise was deafening. For the remainder of my visit that day I hardly ever took my fingers out of my ears.

In the enormous pressroom seven printing presses, each as big as a two-story house, were pounding away, printing sixty thousand copies of the *Daily News* an hour. These vast two-storied Rube Goldberg affairs were a mind-boggling collection of wheels, struts, rollers, and chains, into one end of which giant rolls of blank white paper were fed, eventually to be spat out in the form of finished newspapers at the other end.

Regardless of how far I stuffed my fingers into my eardrums, I simply could not shut out the sound of those presses. And the sound was not just in my ears, for the thundering rumble that rose up from the wood and concrete floor went straight up my legs and through my spine. I imagined this was what it would be like to be standing on an African plain, with a thousand elephants running past me in fear of their lives.

From work station to work station my father led me, showing off his son to each of his colleagues.

While the presses were running, the deaf pressmen wore newspaper hats on their hair (to protect them from the mist of ink that rose off the presses) and smiles of a job well done on their faces. Their hearing co-workers, cotton wadding plugged into their ears, wore matching newspaper hats on their heads but pained expressions on their faces. Now I understood why my father and his deaf pals had been hired, and were valued, by Captain Patterson.

When the presses shuddered to a stop and the last copy of the day's newspaper came down the conveyer belt, my father waved goodbye to his co-workers in the pressroom and marched me off to the composing room, which was where he worked. This huge space housed row upon row upon row of chattering linotype machines, manned by row upon row of workers. Here there was a different sound. Unlike the rolling rumble of panicked elephants in the pressroom, the composing room was filled with the sound of metal clanging on metal, which brought to mind a jungle crowded with monkeys in full cry. Back into my ears went my fingers.

The workers stood shoulder to shoulder, their nimble fingers extracting lead-font type from the drawers of waist-high metal cases, manipulating them with great dexterity into steel frames. Every so often a lead slug containing a group of words, or an advertisement that had been produced on a linotype machine, was dropped in alongside the loose letters of type. When the "page" was completed, the whole affair was locked into place with a metal key.

This was where my father stood five days a week, year after year, from the beginning to the end of his working life. Hunched over his work station, eyeshades protecting his eyes from the murderous glare of the overhead fluorescent strips of light, my father labored, turning lead-type letters into words and sentences. He loved his work.

Pushing me in front of him, he led me forward to meet his deaf pals, who immediately stopped their work and greeted me with warmth, each vying for my attention by making large exaggerated signs. My father told me later that his deaf friends were comparing my signing ability with that of their own children of a similar age. He told me I had done well in their eyes, as some of them had children who didn't sign very proficiently. This was usually the case with the second child (in those days two kids was the norm), because that child was not required to be the family interpreter. The exception, he explained, was when the second child was a girl, as girls tended to be better signers than boys. (My father told my mother that night, when he recapped the day for her, that Myron had received a great compliment from his pals—he signed like a girl. Seeing my father's hands sign "same as a girl," my brother laughed out loud. I, on the other hand, found no humor in the "compliment.")

Meeting my father's hearing co-workers was another matter entirely. These were men who had never once exchanged a meaningful sentence with my deaf father in all the years they had stood side by side in this room. I politely shook every hand offered, but some of the comments I heard, when I removed my fingers from my ears so as to shake those rough hands, echo in my mind to this day. To my face the men said, "Nice to meet you, kid. How come you can hear?" And "How do you like having a deaf father?" "Why does your father talk funny?" "Did your father ever go to school?" And one man even asked me, "Did your father become deaf because his mother dropped him on his head?" This guy wasn't kidding.

My father, oblivious to these questions, proudly beamed down at me as he saw my small hand engulfed in the large hands of his "pals." And that was bad enough, as far as I was concerned.

But what I heard when we walked away, and people spoke behind our backs, as though I too were unable to hear, remains seared into the walls of my mind. "Look at the dummy's kid. He looks normal." "Lou has a nice-looking kid. I wonder why." "Hey, look at that, the dummy's kid. He can talk good." "Would you believe it? The dummy has a kid who can talk." Even then I knew enough to be ashamed of my shame, but I could not overcome it.

Many, many years later, just before my father died, he told me that he knew quite well what his hearing co-workers at the *New York Daily News* really thought of him.

But for that one shining afternoon my father was a proud man, proud in his love of his work, and proud of his son, his firstborn son whom he loved with all his heart.

Memorabilia

Gone Fishing

In memory, I see my father's arms. They were strong arms that ended in equally strong printer's hands, topped off with sensitive, surprisingly slender printer's fingers: fingers that could delicately select assorted loose lead-font type and insert it onto his typestick to create words and sentences that he loaded into a "chase," a steel frame that would comprise a single page of the next day's newspaper. His deft fingers would then lock in the loose type with a key called a "quoin."

These fingers also knew well how to tie a trout fly and how to thread a live worm onto a fishhook so delicately that the worm moved as if it were still burrowing in the dark warm earth until the instant a fish informed it otherwise.

"We're going fishing," my father signed one day, his fingers flapping back and forth like a salmon swimming upstream.

It was my birthday, and he presented me with a bamboo fishing pole as my present.

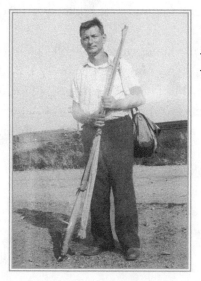

My father with fishing gear: looking for the Big One

A fishing pole? In Brooklyn?

Placing it reverentially in my small hands, his hands met my skepticism with a command: "Practice!"

Practice? In Brooklyn?

For a week I hung my new fishing pole out my third-floor bedroom window, practicing my casting. When I had my cast down well, I dropped the hook outside Mrs.

Abromovitz's kitchen window, one floor below. I had baited it with a peanut butter and jelly sandwich. I pretended she was a tuna. I had read somewhere that tuna like peanut butter and jelly. But Mrs. Abromovitz didn't bite.

I had better luck trolling for the various pieces of clothing, including bloomers that looked like white blimps, strung out on the clothesline that stretched across the alley from her kitchen window to her bathroom window.

I got very good at hooking her brassieres. They were enormous contraptions. Attached by wooden clothespins, they hung down from their sagging straps like two baseball catcher's mitts.

Early one morning my father woke me. Still sleepy, holding his hand, I walked with him to the subway train that would take us to Sheepshead Bay. The bouncing of the train and the screeching wheels did not wake me as I slept, head in my father's lap. We arrived at our stop with a jolt, bouncing me awake.

My father held my hand as we walked toward the ocean, which I could smell but couldn't yet see.

In the darkness we came to the end of Brooklyn and walked up a ramp onto a boat that bobbed up and down, while rocking back and forth at the same time. This could be trouble, I thought.

My father placed my hands on the iron rail and held my shoulders. Feeling his hands holding me in the dark, I was not afraid.

As the sky began to lighten, the engine roared to life, with a puttering cough and the stink of gasoline, and the boat churned away from the dock in a cloud of black exhaust, heading out to sea. Suddenly the sun popped up at the edge of the ocean like a silhouette at a Coney Island shooting gallery, and I could see our wake stretching far behind, all the way back to Brooklyn. Seagulls followed, yelling down at us, "We're hungry. What's for lunch?" Boy, were they ever going to be disappointed when we caught all their food.

The boat stopped, and the captain dropped the anchor. As the sky began to brighten on the horizon, my father breathed deeply of the salt air, turned to me, and said, "Let's catch a fish for dinner. A big one!"

I baited my hook. We fished all morning. We caught nothing. After a quick lunch we dropped our baited hooks back into the sea. We fished some more, all that afternoon, with the same result. We caught no fish.

As the sun began to sink over New Jersey, and the light began to fade, our captain pulled up the anchor and pointed the boat back toward Brooklyn. My father's hands never left the railing; they had nothing to say. But his face said it all.

On the way to the subway station to catch the train that would take us home, my father stopped and bought a fish. A very large fish.

"If you don't say anything," he signed, "neither will I."

When we arrived at our apartment door, he put the fish, wrapped in newspaper, into my arms and rang the bell that activated a flashing light in our hallway and a lamp in our living room.

My mother and my brother were happy to see us.

"Hoo-ha-ha, my husband, Lou, and my son the fisherman," she signed, and took the big dead fish to the kitchen. My mother always referred to my father as "my husband, Lou," not "your father."

She did this unconsciously. Her immediate world, her self-contained silent world, was her husband, Lou, and herself. They were the binary stars of their own silent cosmos.

My brother and I were two close planets in tight orbit. I knew with all my being that she loved us, but we were different because we could hear. Their hearing parents and siblings were in orbits farther distant. As were neighbors, then fellow workers. And finally, like all the visible but distant stars in the universe, came the vast multitude of hearing people whom they could never possibly know.

"Your husband, Lou?" I would sometimes ask her, in my poor attempt at humor. "Who is *that*? Sounds like my father."

My mother looked at me as if I had lost my mind. For my deaf mother, in the hierarchy of her emotions and allegiance, *her husband* came before *my father*.

That night, after my mother with the care of a brain surgeon carefully removed every single bone for my brother (I was old enough to fend for myself), we ate the fish. My mother kept looking at me with every bite she took, a smile on her face. As for my brother, he acted as if I had caught a whale.

I felt a little guilty that they believed that I had caught the fish. But only a little. The fish was delicious, bones and all.

8

The Smell of Reading

*O*nce a month, on a Saturday afternoon, as regular as clock-work, my father, with great ceremony, took my mother, my brother, and me to the local Chinese restaurant for lunch. Eating out was a very big deal in those tail-end days of the Depression; the economic benefits of America's fighting a world war had not, as yet, trickled down to our corner of the world, our peaceful Brooklyn neighborhood.

We would dress up for this occasion, I in my newest R. and H. Macy's suit, my brother in the latest fashion for small kids, my mother in her best dress, topped with her fox stole, and my father in his tweed suit. ("I look like a professor," he always signed, meer-schaum pipe smoldering away in one corner of his mouth. His model was Robert Donat in *Goodbye, Mr. Chips,* a movie he favored, even though he could never quite figure out what the actors were up to.)

Once my father had examined my brother and me for stray hairs, unnoticed stains, and scuffed shoe leather, we descended in the elevator to the ground floor. After a final careful look at each of us, my father pushed open the heavy ornate glass lobby door, and we exited, linked together in a line, my parents arm in arm at the center, I holding my father's hand, my brother holding my mother's hand, all heading toward Kings Highway. As we walked up our block, eyes straight ahead, we would be closely watched by every one of our neighbors, who behind my back made their un-failingly unchanged comments: "Considering they're deaf-mutes, they dress well." "See how nice the deafies dress their boys." "The father's a deaf-mute, but he has a good job." "The dummies are taking their kids to the 'Chinks.'"

This last was, sadly, an all-too-common term in our neighbor-hood, generally used by us Jews, the same people who were ap-palled when the Irish in the Red Hook section of Brooklyn called *them* "Yids." And as if that were not irony enough, even to my young ears, these were the same people who publicly objected to the treatment the Chinese had experienced in Manchuria at the hands, and bayonets, of Japanese soldiers, who were of course known as "Japs." Anyway, I reasoned, in some small though mis-guided attempt at rationalization, this circle of unthinking preju-dice was large and inclusive; no one was immune. The Irish *and* the Jews called the Polish "Polacks"; the Polish called the Italians "Wops"; the Italians called the Irish "Micks"; and the Irish called the Chinese "Chinks." Thus the circle of casual discrimination was complete.

What the Chinese called all of us, I had no idea.

As for the neighbors' use of the term "dummies," I had heard it from an early age, but it seemed somehow worse to me than the ethnic epithets because those words were group names, whereas "dummy" was personal; it referred specifically to the only deaf people the neighbors knew, my father and my mother. Nonetheless I was numb, if only from constant exposure to it, and did not allow it to interfere with my enjoyment of our monthly family outing.

The Chinese restaurant was located on the ground floor of a row of connected two-story wooden buildings. The street-level spaces were all filled with shops: bakery, poultry, hardware, vegetable, pharmacy, barber, beauty, and of course the neighborhood candy store.

As far as I was concerned, the highlight of this eating-out ritual was the sight of my father conversing in broken gestures with our Chinese waiter, while he in turn responded in broken English. Both of them studiously navigated their way through the dense, food-stained menu, filled with columns of incomprehensible Chinese characters, alongside garbled English translations. The waiter screamed good-naturedly at my father the contents of the day's specialty of the house, as if sheer volume alone could get my father to *hear* the description of that delicacy. My father would just as loudly *scream* his gestures of approval right back at the waiter. Their heads nodding in perfect smiling agreement during this astonishing performance, neither one of them had any idea what the other was saying.

As for me, what would otherwise have been a situation of stinging embarrassment was rendered funny, as the other diners were regulars and were quite used to this scene. It was clear to me that they were staring at our table not in disgust but in tolerant amusement. I would settle for that.

One Saturday we had our usual Chinese lunch, beginning with the specialty of the house (it was always the same, month after month), an inedible, bone-laden, soggy bleached white fish with the most amazing pair of bulging sightless eyes staring at me in mute accusation. This was followed by two choices from column A (always the same choices, month after month) and one from column B (ditto), washed down with an undrinkable, thinly colored green liquid filled with floating black flecks. The meal concluded, as it always did, with a fortune cookie, the message of which, much prized and heartily laughed over by my father and mother, made absolutely no sense to me, although I liked the taste of the cookie itself.

But this day there was a change in the ritual.

After a close study of the bill, minutely itemized but thoroughly incomprehensible except for the total cost, my father paid and then turned to me and signed, "You can read now. It's time for you to get a library card."

Above the Chinese restaurant was our local library. I had heard about this place from the older kids, but I had never set foot there, since you needed a library card to enter, as I had been told (warned) by the big kids. They said the place contained every book that had ever been printed in the whole world. I had no idea if this was true. *Every book?* Why, there must be hundreds of them, I thought. Having just learned to read really well, I was more than idly curious as to the truth of the matter: *every* book? But then, the older kids could not be trusted. Most everything they told us, every warning they solemnly uttered, turned out to be greatly overblown.

My father and mother were great readers. Being deaf, they went to books as their main source of daily entertainment. Our little apartment was filled with books, books of all kinds. Some books were filled with pictures of far-off places depicting pyramids, camels, endless sand deserts, giant rivers, high waterfalls, deep canyons, strange beasts, and sailing ships. I especially loved the pictures of wooden-hulled, canvas-masted, cannonade-sided sailing vessels breaking, oaken shouldered, through giant frothy waves. And now that I had learned to read what the words under these pictures said, I had been dreaming of having a library card of my very own—a dream that was now about to be realized.

Exiting the Chinese restaurant, we made a hard right and

entered an adjacent door leading to a steep flight of well-trod wooden stairs.

At the top of the stairs was a painted glass door proclaiming, "Brooklyn Public Library." Pushing it open, my father led us into a single large room. The first thing I noticed was that it was filled, end to end, top to bottom, with *every* book that had ever been printed in the whole world. The second was that the place smelled like a Chinese restaurant. (The library was just above the restaurant kitchen.)

I could hardly believe that the hundreds of books lining the shelves were free for the asking. As a child of the Depression, I had been drilled in the sure knowledge that everything had a price. *Everything.* The idea that merely by presenting a library card—nothing more than a piece of cardboard—I would be allowed to remove these precious books seemed inconceivable.

At first I found the trust placed in me near to overwhelming. I would examine every single page of a book with the care of a brain surgeon before I would dream of checking it out. If there was even a single crease at the corner of a page—or, horrors, a food stain somewhere on the page—I would bring that blemish to the attention of the librarian. And she would note on the flyleaf, in her spidery handwriting, "Peanut butter stain? Pg. 36." Or all too commonly, "Underlining. Pg. 12." Even now, many decades later, I still find myself flipping through the pages of a library book, prior to checkout, to ascertain its condition.

What I found most miraculous about the library was the sheer quantity of words to be found in the seemingly endless army of books marching shoulder to shoulder, row upon row, on the shelves. Words. Words. Words. Written words. Preserved words. The library was a warehouse of words. Words to decipher. Words to learn. Words to add to my vocabulary. Words to make mine.

The words found in books were in sharp contrast to the words of my first language. Sign is a live, contemporaneous, visual-gestural language and consists of hand shapes, hand positioning, facial expressions, and body movements. Simply put, it is for me the most beautiful, immediate, and expressive of languages, because it incorporates the entire human body. In the case of sign, a picture truly is worth a thousand words. The signs of my father and mother went from their hands and faces and bodies directly into my consciousness. Thus as a child I never perceived language as a series of discrete units that added up to thoughts. Instead, I absorbed meaning whole, all at once, through my eyes.

Printed words were another matter entirely, and as I came to learn more and more of them, I discovered their unique charms. When reading a book, I could linger over every word, and sound it out in my mind for the sheer pleasure it gave me. Each word was like a musical note and could be enjoyed both for its own sake and for the sound it made as it combined with an adjoining word. Best of all was the melody I heard in a perfect sentence. This was a language of the mind; sign was a language of the heart. Sign was a beautiful painting, absorbed whole, evoking emotion along with meaning. Written language—my second language—was a language that required the brain for translation.

Reading was to become the passion of my life, our local branch of the Brooklyn Library my childhood refuge. Armed with a library card, I could escape to this quiet sanctuary anytime I became overwhelmed by the demands that my father placed on me. Here in this musty, sweet-smelling place, filled with the faint odor of soy sauce, I could open a book and be magically transported to the ends of the earth.

And so I came to spend ever-increasing amounts of time in that library, surrounded by all the words I could ever hope to learn, listening to the music of those words in my mind, all the while enveloped in the comforting scent of Chinese food.

To this day I often find myself taking an exploratory sniff at a library book, as though in expectation that a faint odor of chow mein will rise off the pages.

9

Falling in Love

I fell in love for the first time in the second grade. Actually, I didn't so much *fall* in love as choose, pragmatically, to *be* in love. (This would not be the case in later life, as I have been married three times in all—certainly I am more optimistic than pragmatic.)

On the first day of school I spotted a new girl in our class. Our desks were arranged alphabetically, and as I was a *U,* I sat in the rear of the room, while she, a *W,* sat at a desk to my right, immediately under a window. My earliest memory of her is the glowing halo that ringed her golden curls as a beam of sunlight fell on her head. She looked like an angel. Her small, straight nose was flecked with freckles, and completing the picture, her generous, ever-smiling mouth was filled with tiny, unbelievably white teeth.

Not until she stood up at her desk for the first time, having been called on by the teacher to read a poem, did I realize that she was much taller than me. And in all the years we traveled from grade to grade, ever upward, right into and through high school, I never caught up. She turned out to be the tallest child in our class and in every class she was ever in. Her name was Eve.

The second thing I noticed about Eve that day was her left hand.

Actually, what I noted was the absence of her left hand, as she kept it in her lap the entire hour. And when she stood to read, she pushed it deep into the pocket of her tartan dress. This seemed odd to me, and awkward, as it meant that she had to hold the heavy book of poems she was reading from with only one hand.

A week of classes passed before the mystery was solved. One morning she sneezed. She was dipping her pen in the inkwell of her desk with her right hand when the sneeze overcame her, so reflexively she brought her left hand to her mouth. It was then that I saw that her left pinky curled over the adjacent finger. The pinky looked like the shepherd's crook in a picture book I had read.

Eve saw me staring at her hand and quickly dropped it into her lap, where it lay hidden beneath her desktop. Staring straight ahead, with a fixed expression on her face, she blushed. I saw that she was embarrassed.

As the school year progressed, I noticed that the other children also became aware of Eve's hand. Like children the world over, instinctive in their cruelty, they would stare at her hand whenever it made a rare appearance. And they would laugh at the sight of it. Eve would cringe at their stares and shrink at the sound of their laughter. She never stood straight, as she tried to minimize her height. But when her classmates laughed, she didn't just slump; she seemed almost to hunch over. Often the laughter was not even directed at her. Kids laugh at most anything. But for Eve, every single laugh was directed at her and her misshapen hand.

Whenever I saw her distress, at some deep level of my young soul I instinctively related to what she was feeling because I had my own source of shame that, like hers, had to do with feeling different. For children, anything that marks them out as different is acutely embarrassing. In my case it was my father and mother who were different, and I was ashamed of them, in the same way that Eve was ashamed of her hand.

Once I made the connection between her embarrassment and mine, I decided to be in love with her.

It took some time, but after a while Eve became comfortable in my presence. Though she lived just around the corner from me, on West Tenth Street, in those days, at our age, *around the corner* was another world altogether. We children on West Ninth Street had no need to ever leave our block. There was absolutely nothing on West Tenth Street that was not available to me right outside our apartment house door on West Ninth Street—until I met Eve. Soon I was carrying her books home for her at the end of every school day. And I arranged to meet her at the stoop in front of her two-family house every morning before school began.

Eventually Eve introduced me to her mother. She had no father. The reason for this absence of a father was never made clear to me. And was never discussed.

After some time had passed, I asked Eve to come to my house. She agreed, and I duly introduced her to my mother. Just as she never said anything about her absent father, I had not told Eve that my mother was deaf. I didn't know how. And somehow I knew that it wouldn't matter to Eve.

Although surprised at my signing to my mother as I introduced her, Eve did not stare or act funny in any way. Afterward she asked me many questions: "How did you learn sign language?" "How did you communicate with your parents before you learned?" "Have they always been deaf?" "Why aren't you deaf as well?" Her questions seemed born of genuine interest and did not embarrass me.

I had some questions of my own. "Were you born that way?" "Did you get your hand caught in a door?" "Can a doctor straighten out your pinky?" My questions did not embarrass her either.

In time she asked me to teach her some signs. As most signs require two hands to execute, she had some difficulty at first. But eventually she lost her self-consciousness in front of me and learned even the most complex ones I taught her. Using both of her hands, she would show off her signing to my mother. My mother would sign back, "Very clear. Very beautiful signs." And I would translate my mother's approval to Eve.

One day our teacher told the class that every morning of the following month we would begin the day with a student doing a demonstration of some kind of learning project. The project was ours to choose. Our teacher suggested some possible projects for our consideration. We could prepare a science project, for instance, involving butterflies in a jar. As she said this, every kid had the identical thought: *Butterflies in Brooklyn?* Groans of protest spread throughout the classroom. "Or possibly you could show us worms burrowing into their habitat." But where would we find worms? Practically all of Brooklyn was paved over with concrete and macadam. More groans. "Or you could make an ant farm." Finally, we thought, here at last was a practical suggestion. After all, we knew where to find ants on our block. But we couldn't all present ant farms.

Having exhausted her limited repertory of ideas, our teacher gave up and said, "*Any* project will be satisfactory." She added, "Originality, and mastery of the project, is what counts. Make it interesting. And if you wish, you may pair up and present the project jointly."

I looked at Eve, and Eve looked at me. In unspoken agreement we agreed we would join forces to prepare and present a project. But what would the project be?

After much discussion in the lunchroom, we hit upon an idea. An excellent idea, we thought. It would be original, as the teacher insisted. It would be interesting—of that we were sure. Now all we had to do was master it; or at least Eve would have to, since we had decided to do a sign language project. We would call our project "Writing on Air."

For the next four weeks Eve and I spent most of our spare time after school practicing signing on her front stoop. We were so energetic, we drew a crowd of fascinated neighborhood kids.

"Teach us! Teach us!" they clamored. "We want to learn your secret language."

I, who had always been somewhat embarrassed to sign to my father on the street, now exulted in the attention my knowledge of this exotic form of communication was garnering. And so I began to show off, flaunting with exaggerated gestures some of the more complicated signs that my father had taught me. Of course the signs I enacted were basically just a vocabulary list presented for effect alone—I made no attempt to use them in context. But that didn't seem to matter. What mattered was the complexity and dexterity of the sign itself.

My sign for *acrobat* brought down the house. My father had recently taken me to the Ringling Brothers Circus at Madison Square Garden and had taught me many circus signs. They were all new to me, as we had had no previous need for them in our Brooklyn apartment. Once I learned them, however, I found any excuse to use them. "Look, Mom," I signed as I jumped onto my bed. "I'm an *acrobat*." My right index and middle fingers, shaped like the legs of an acrobat, stood on my open, upturned left palm. Then the "legs" on my right hand flexed, jumped, flipped over, and executed a double somersault before descending back onto my left palm, where they stood, triumphant, slightly quivering from the impact. My sign was so good, I swear you could see the sawdust covering the circus arena of my left palm. At least I could— and my mother applauded.

As for *secret* signs, far and away the best one was the graphic sign for *defecate*. The right thumb is grasped in the fist of the left hand. Then quickly—or as the case may be when somewhat constipated, with exquisite slowness—the thumb is drawn down from the enclosed right fist. Faster would be the case if you had been eating prunes.

The children loved it! Now every kid in the neighborhood could say *shit* in sign.

Finally the day arrived as scheduled. The presenting of the projects began.

Eve and I sat through the most boring displays and incomprehensible explanations of why fireflies light up (which they absolutely refused to do in their jelly jar homes, being otherwise occupied sucking on the grape jelly under the lid); where mosquitoes go to die after biting you (this display featured ten dead mosquitoes lying peacefully on a bed of leaves at the bottom of an airless jar whose lid a kid had neglected to puncture with a nail); and how a moth turns into a butterfly (this one we didn't believe for a minute). Then it was our turn.

We stood at the front of the class. The idea was that Eve would position herself somewhat to my rear, where I couldn't see her, and she would hold up—in her right hand, of course—a drawing of the sign I was supposed to perform. When she called out the word for the sign, I would, from memory, execute it, in a kind of visual spelling bee.

When the teacher introduced us, half the class made the sign for *shit*. The other half nearly fell out of their chairs laughing. The teacher stood, dumbstruck, not having a clue as to what was going on. The room was a bedlam of hands in motion.

Shit, shit, shit signs flew through the air, were flung through the air. It was a hailstorm of shit. A tornado of turds.

It took quite a while for the teacher to restore order.

Once again she introduced Eve and me, with the warning that any further outburst, whatever the heck it was about, would be rewarded with a trip to the principal's office.

We began. Eve called out "penguin." I dropped both my hands, palms facing downward, fingers held together, to either side of my waist. Then, hunching up my shoulders, I alternately raised and lowered each shoulder. To emphasize this sign, I lurched forward, stiff-legged, mimicking the lumbering gait of a penguin as it traversed an ice floe. The class applauded.

Eve asked for "deer." Now I made what I imagined was the face of a startled deer, possibly caught in the headlights of a car on Flatbush Avenue, placing both my open hands above my head, all ten fingers splayed and shooting outward into stiff antler appendages. These I wiggled convincingly, as the class broke into a cheer.

"Elk?"

I was an elk.

"Moose?"

I was a moose.

The class loved it. "More. More!"

"Elephant?" My right hand formed a cup with its back resting against my nose. My hand moved gracefully, ponderously, out from my nose, curving downward, and while it turned under, seeking peanuts that were now visible to the imagination, on the dirt floor of the circus ring of our minds.

The class erupted in shouts of glee. My signs were killing them. This had to be better than ten dead mosquitoes and a bunch of fireflies that would not light.

Eve took me through a jungle of animals and a zoo full of exotic birds.

Then she began a list of the more complex signs that we had agreed upon.

The first sign was for a concept we were both familiar with. "What is the sign for *embarrass?*" she asked.

I made the sign for *red,* as in blood, moving my index finger up and down my red lips; then both my palms cradled my face, moving slowly upward, as if the red blush of blood were rising up, suffusing my entire face in a blossoming blush of mortification.

The class was fascinated.

Then Eve asked, "What is the sign for *discard?*" I drew a blank. I stood mute.

Eve prompted again: "*Discard?*"

I stood there at the front of the class, all eyes focused on me, my hands at my sides, defeated, a genuine blush of embarrassment now flooding my face; somehow I had completely forgotten this sign.

Eve realized that there was no use in asking me again to sign this concept.

She dropped the cards and rushed to my side to rescue me.

Discard is a sign that requires both hands to execute.

Without a moment's hesitation, she withdrew her left hand from her pocket and positioned it in the air for the entire class to see. Palm open and facing the class, pinky finger crooked in its permanently twisted position, with her open "normal" right hand she drew her fingertips across the palm of her hated left hand toward her pinky.

Suddenly she closed her right hand, as if clasping something, and swiftly withdrew it from her left palm, as if she had discovered a loathsome object there, and with a forceful motion she flung it to the floor, all the while making an expression of such distaste that the class fully expected the obscene object to leap up and scurry out of the room.

The audience was stunned into silence at her performance. The children fully understood what Eve had done, what her sign had signified—for her.

No one laughed.

Suddenly the class erupted in shouts of approval. Now Eve blushed, not in embarrassment, but from pride.

From that day on she never hid her hand again.

And at that moment I fell genuinely, not calculatingly, in love with Eve.

10
Tales Told

*O*ne afternoon after school was out, a sudden drenching downpour drove all of the kids on my block back into their apartments. As was her habit whenever she saw me house-bound and at loose ends, my mother pulled me into the kitchen, sat me down at the table, and proceeded to cook me something to eat. I loved to watch her cook: throw in a little bit of this, a little bit of that, then a pinch of something else (never consulting a recipe, never measuring), mix, turn up the flame on the stove, and then wait until the mouthwatering concoction was done, which she always knew intuitively, without once looking at the clock.

Setting before me a fresh batch of matzoh brei, she watched me eat, with the strangest expression on her face.

"You know, your father was not my first choice for a husband," she signed.

As good as the delightful mix of crumbly eggs and cracking-crisp matzoh was, I stopped eating. *What in the world,* I thought, *is this all about?*

"I want to tell you a story," she signed. "I want you to understand me."

I put down my fork and concentrated on my mother's hands and face and body. And I listened to her voice as she signed. My friends could not understand my mother's speech, but I understood every word.

"When I was a girl, as you know, I loved going to the beach in Coney Island. It was my favorite place in the whole world, outside of my school. I was a naughty girl. I liked boys. I was *crazy* about boys. And they were *crazy* about me."

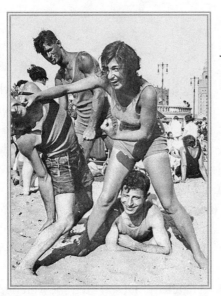

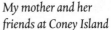

My mother and her friends at Coney Island

There are many signs for *crazy,* but the one she used to indicate how she loved those young boys involved her kissing the back of her closed hand. Over and over she kissed her hand, indicating clearly the strength of her feelings, her need for acceptance, her desire for attention.

To convey to me the power she had over them, she shaped her

hand in a claw and shook it back and forth in front of her face, indicating that they were *crazy/dizzy/nuts* for her.

Then she told me the story of her great lost love.

"My big love was a hearing boy. I loved him, and he adored me."

Describing this Coney Island Adonis, long since consigned to the mists of memory, but re-created in her mind this day as vividly as if he still waited for her on Bay 6, she spoke of him lovingly and in great detail. He had a golden tan, she said, the result of repeated exposures to the summer sun, aided by the hourly application to his skin of a concoction of chicken fat, virgin olive oil, and iodine. "When I looked at him," she signed, a faraway look in her eyes, "his skin glowed, and I saw his body covered in a golden light."

Apparently he lifted weights, for she told me he had muscles all over his body, even in places she didn't think boys *could* have muscles. When she said this, I could swear, she blushed.

"My father hated him," she signed. "He had heard about this boy from a neighbor, who told my father that this boy was touching me and kissing me under the boardwalk. This was not true. But I knew he wanted to do that, if I'd let him. I was a flirt. I was a tease. I was naughty. But I was a good girl." She smiled, no doubt picturing in her mind the beautiful, fresh, innocent young girl she had been so many summers ago. Then her face darkened.

"One day when I came home from the beach, my father slapped me across the face. I was shocked. My father had *never* hit me. My father, Max, was a Gypsy, you know. My mother told me that his family lived in the forest in the old country. 'They lived like animals,' she said. I don't think my mother ever loved my father.

"Though he was free with his hands with my brothers, he had always spoiled me. We had no money, and he had no steady job, but what little he had, he would spend on me, buying me small treats. I think he felt sad all of his life that I was deaf. He didn't know why, but he blamed himself. He felt guilty.

"It was only after he slapped me that I found out the reason for his anger. The boy I was crazy for didn't have a job. And didn't have a trade. And he was *not* deaf. Just like baseball, three strikes and you're out.

"My father forbade me to see the boy ever again. And the next weekend he went to Bay 6 and confronted the boy, muscles and all. When the boy laughed in my father's face, at his arm-waving and screaming, my father, who was strong as an ox, socked him.

"From then on the boy paid no attention to me. I was heartbroken, especially when I saw him flirting with another deaf girl. I don't know if I really loved him or not, but what I needed, I realized later, was the attention he gave me. Attention from a hearing person, which no other hearing person had ever shown me."

I was amazed at this story. I knew next to nothing about my grandfather Max. The idea that he was a Gypsy fascinated me, especially since the only Gypsies I had ever seen were the ones in the movie *The Wolfman*. And in that movie they were a strange, evil-looking people, rattling around in the forest in their horse-drawn wagons. And of course the idea of my mother as a young girl, in love with someone other than my father, was almost inconceivable to me.

My mother continued her story. "My father then put out the word in the deaf community of New York: *Find me a deaf man for my deaf daughter. I only ask that he have a trade. That he have a job. That he is not a bum.* And he added, *A union card would be a plus.*"

I couldn't help but wonder who I would have been if my mother had married that hearing boy. What would it have been like, I thought, to have lived in a home divided right down the middle by one silent and one hearing parent? I simply could not imagine such a thing and was glad that my grandfather, Max the Gypsy, had socked the boy with the golden skin all these many years ago. Besides, I loved my father and could not for a minute imagine having any other one but him.

"That's how I met Lou. At first I didn't love him, like I thought I loved that boy. But I didn't know what love was, when I was a girl. And when the nurse put you in my arms, just after you were born, I knew I had made the right decision."

Then my mother came around the table, kissed me, and signed, "Eat!"

Memorabilia

What's in a Name

On my street Paul Abruzzi's nickname was Paulie; Frank was known as Frankie; Thomas, Tommy; John, Johnny; Ronald, Ronnie; and my pal Harold was called Heshie. I was the one kid on my block whose name, Myron, could not readily be turned into a nickname. But that didn't stop my friends from giving me one: Mike—and then, of course, Mikey.

My mother would have been horrified, not to mention deeply offended, if she had known that I had abandoned what was, to her deaf ears, the beautiful-sounding name she had selected for me: *Myron.*

But deaf parents typically create their own nicknames for their children, as it would be quite tedious and unnecessarily time-consuming to finger-spell every letter of a child's name when seeking his attention or talking with him. Thus they give their children names that can be conveniently—

and succinctly—signed. Such nicknames are known as name-signs.

A name-sign is not lightly decided upon. After all, this will be the way the parent addresses the child for the rest of his childhood—and often for the rest of his life.

My mother loved the name Myron so much that she wanted it to be recalled in my name-sign. So her first attempt at creating one for me involved using the initials of my name, M and U. My mother reasoned that MU must sound like the noise that cows make—MOO. Looking at me one day, she shaped her hands into an approximation of a cow's horns by curling the three middle fingers inward to the palm and extending the thumb and pinky. These *horns* she placed on the sides of her head, thumbs touching her temples, and twisted them forward while sounding out in her deaf voice, MOOOO. "M.y.r.o.n.," she finger-spelled. "How do you like this name?"

I didn't!

One morning as I was about to run downstairs to play, my mother stopped me in my tracks and signed, "Wait! I have a new name for you." The deaf believe that the ideal name-sign for a child should encapsulate in one visual gesture the very essence of the child. My mother's second idea for a name-sign must have seemed to her like a no-brainer. She was sure that it truly captured the nature of her beloved child—the boy who seemed most comfortable high up on the limb of a tree or climbing walls. She looked into my eyes and began to scratch her sides repeatedly—which, of course, is the sign for *monkey*.

Needless to say, I rejected this name-sign, too. I did not want my mother coming up to me, while I was playing in the street with my friends, and addressing me with the sign for *monkey.*

Unable to find a name-sign that I would accept, my mother went back to the way she had addressed me since she named me as a baby—*MHHHAAARINNN.*

$\mathcal{A}$ll of my life I never cared for my given name. I preferred to be known as Mike. My present wife, my two former wives, my three children, my grandchildren, my business associates, teammates, and friends, and even my bank all know me as Mike. In fact, when I left my deaf home, I ceased to be Myron to anyone except my parents. However, one day when talking with my mother—who had come to live with me at the age of eighty-nine, when she could no longer take care of herself—I summoned up the nerve to ask her why it was that she had named me Myron.

My deaf mother, who could not hear a sound, did not hesitate for an instant: "Because it *sounds* so beautiful."

One day I received an advance copy of my first children's book. I immediately showed it to my mother. Holding it lovingly on her lap as if it were a live thing and not just a book, she slowly traced my name with her finger, while a broad smile spread across her face. "Beautiful," she signed. "MHHHAAARINNN," she said.

I've preferred being called Myron ever since.

11

The Sound of Color

In those halcyon early days of public education, long before children would be held strictly accountable to a national testing demanded by a government that acknowledged little accountability for itself, public schools in Brooklyn routinely offered a class in arts and crafts. I, who had no artistic ability whatsoever, would bring home every week a crinkled sheet of sketch paper covered in indecipherable scrawls, with occasional splotches of color. And I, like every one of my classmates, no doubt, would be routinely commended by my teacher, and lavishly praised by my parents, for my "work of art."

One day I showed my father a sketch I had done which, I explained—since an explanation seemed necessary—represented the Brooklyn Bridge.

"And here are the seagulls." I pointed proudly at a tangle of black lines.

"Yes," my father's hands tentatively said. "I think I see them."

Hanging over the tortured mess, I had colored in a red circle. A very red circle. It was the one spot of color on the entire page, my artistic sensibilities being quite cramped.

"And that's the sun," I signed with exaggerated imagination. "I call this 'Morning in Brooklyn.'"

My father stared at the red circle. "Red," he told me, "is an angry color. It sounds loud. Very loud. So loud that it sometimes hurts my ears."

As I said, my father thought color had sound. I thought this strange, since my father was deaf and could hear no sound at all.

"Why do you think that?" I once asked him.

"In school I saw a painting of a man holding his ears. In the noisy picture the man was screaming. Above him the sky was an angry, swirling red color. I never forgot that painting."

"Blue was a cool color," he said, fanning his face. "Like water and must sound wet."

I couldn't begin to imagine what my father meant. Wet? What did *wet* sound like, anyway?

Hardly a day went by that my father did not find an occasion to ask me what a color sounded like.

"How does the color black sound?" he asked me one summer day as we were walking on Surf Avenue in Coney Island. It was the middle of August, and we were on our way to the beach. Above us gray storm clouds were gathering. They filled the sky. They were beginning to bump into each other. Where they merged, the gray blended into black. And where they piled up, one massive black cloud upon another, they turned an even darker shade of black. A cold salt-laden breeze suddenly swept down Surf Avenue from the direction of Nathan's, loaded with the blended smells of grilled franks and mustard, knishes, hot buttered corn, and a subtle suggestion of popcorn.

Day turned into night as lightning split the darkness, followed by claps of thunder. The clouds cracked open, and torrential rain poured from the sky, quickly turning the steaming asphalt into small debris-cluttered rivers, overwhelming the storm drains, then backing them up, causing miniature waves to break across Surf Avenue. The rides emptied and stopped. People ran for cover as the rain fell in wind-driven sheets of water. I tugged on my father's hand, but he stood still, looking up at the blackest sky I had ever seen.

"What does black sound like?" he asked me again.

Thunder loud enough to hurt my ears banged down on my head.

"Like thunder," I signed, repeatedly banging my two fists together.

"I don't understand," he signed, his face pinched in frustration. "What does *thunder* sound like?"

I was desperate. I was soaked. I began to shiver. "Like a hammer," I signed, now raising and lowering my fist, as if I were striking my opposite fist with an invisible hammer.

My father thought about that, his face relaxing into comprehension. "Yes, like a hammer. Hard, like my hands."

Satisfied, he took my hand, and we ran under an awning. The meager trees along the curb bent in the wind. Leaves torn from their thin branches flew all about us.

"I *feel* the wind on my face. Tell me, what is wind sound?" my father demanded.

As I was trying to come up with an answer for my father, the black clouds blew out over the ocean. The Wonder Wheel began to turn again, the empty white cars swinging out over the boardwalk, reflecting golden sunlight.

"Never mind," my father signed. "We'll go to the beach before all the good spots are taken." My mother was home with a cold that day, and my brother was keeping her company. "Say hi to the deafies," she had told me as we went out the door that morning. "And say hi to Ben," she added to my father, her hands laughing.

We were not the first to arrive at the small patch of beach that the deaf had long ago claimed as their very own, the place where they could all be together. Three deaf couples from the Bronx and one from Queens had gotten there before us. They always did, since they did not want to be relegated to the warmer, boardwalk side of the circle that would form and re-form all day long with each new arrival. We added our beach chair to the circle, which immediately expanded to accommodate us.

All morning long the deaf streamed in from every borough in New York. Each addition to the group caused conversations to stop in midair while chairs were lifted and readjusted to enlarge the circle, after which the hands resumed their flights in midsentence, gesturing furiously to one another.

I was intrigued even then by the wild diversity of language on display, the different styles reflecting a wide variety of personalities and geographic origins, as well as differences between the sexes. The men tended to sign more aggressively, more assertively than the women. The outgoing personalities signed expansively, while the shy tended to make smaller, more guarded signs. Some were so reserved that they made only the most tentative gestures in the air, constipated strings of small, stunted signs. Some signed with abandon, even boisterously, while others signed demurely. Some signed loudly, some softly. Some signed with comic exaggeration, while the signing of others was more controlled, more thoughtful. A couple who had moved to the Bronx from a small town in Georgia signed with an accent I didn't recognize. My father told me they signed with a drawl, and it was true that their signs did seem to flow from their hands like syrup, thick and slow.

Strangely, there was one deaf lady who had suffered a stroke many years before who seemed to stutter when she signed. It was as though her signs stuck to her hands. Impatiently, she shook them off her fingers in an attempt to be understood.

One man's signs seemed halting, primitive, even childish. My father caught me staring, with what must have been a puzzled look on my face, and explained.

"When he was a boy, he lived on a farm. He grew up deaf on that farm. He had a big hearing family, but his family had no sign. His family was poor. It was a hard life. His father needed the boy to help with the farm work. Finally the boy went to deaf school when he was fourteen years old. There he learned sign. But it was too late. He never learned good. He is still a little deaf boy in his own mind. Now all the time he talks like a child. Simple. He never gets better. Sad."

My father's signs tended to be quick, impatient, insistent—typical of the signs of the deaf who live in a big city.

Many years later I looked back on that panorama of word-pictures painted in the air above the sand of Coney Island and saw that it was as complex and as colorful in its own way as the ceiling above the Sistine Chapel.

"Where is Sally?" one set of hands asked. (Sally was the nickname by which my mother had been known ever since her teenage days at the Lexington School for the Deaf.) Those hands belonged to Ben from Coney Island. He had been one of my mother's many boyfriends when she was a young girl.

"She's home. My wife, Sarah, has a cold," my father answered, carefully spelling out the name *Sarah* and emphasizing the word *wife*.

My father hated Ben and had never gotten over my mother's long-ago interest in him.

"Sure, he's a good-looking guy," I observed him say one day to Mort, a close friend he'd first met at Fanwood, the deaf school they'd both been sent to as children.

"Sure, he still has all his hair, but I bet it's dyed. And he fools around on his wife, Mary," he added, his hands whispering in small guarded signs so no one else could see what he was signing.

"Ah, Lou, let it go, will you?" Mort signed. "That was fifteen years ago. Who cares? You are a union man, and he's a bum!"

"Easy for you to say," my father answered him.

"My *wife*, Sarah, says hi," he added to Ben, while his grim face belied the pleasant greeting.

Just then four more deaf couples arrived, lugging beach chairs and picnic baskets and beach umbrellas, their kids hanging on for dear life lest they be lost in the commotion.

The circle readjusted to accommodate the newcomers. Down went the beach chairs and up went the hands, fluttering wildly like the wings of a flock of geese taking flight at the sound of a shotgun blast. They had not seen one another since last weekend, and there was much news to tell.

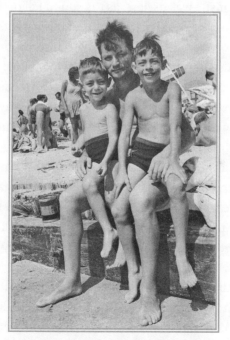

Irwin and I with our father at Coney Island

We kids sat on beach towels in the middle of the ever-expanding circle, like small animals in a human cage made up of our parents, beach chairs, and beach umbrellas, our protection against the possibility of getting lost. To be lost in Coney Island on a Sunday in August was a scary experience for any kid, but especially for a kid whose parents were deaf. When lost (an ever-present danger, since the beach was so crowded), the child would invariably be accosted by an adult sympathetic to the sight of a child crying his heart out, who would take him to the nearest lifeguard station. I say "him" because girls rarely wandered off and got lost in those days. There the lifeguard would ask the kid his name. Armed with that essential information, the lifeguard would dangle the kid over the railing of his elevated perch, while blowing his whistle in a series of ear-splitting screeches. In our case, of course, the whistle was useless, as the sound fell on what were literally deaf ears. We could only hope that our parents would eventually notice we were missing and maybe, just maybe, stop talking to their friends long enough to come looking for us.

By late afternoon, when the last of the arrivals had finally made it, having traveled by ferry and subway all the way from Staten Island, there were well over one hundred beach chairs in a perfect circle. A deaf man or woman occupied each chair. And each man or woman was signing frantically to another man or woman in the circle, sometimes to one clear across the circle, far away.

There were few secrets in the deaf community at Coney Island.

"What do the waves sound like?" my father asked me out of the blue. "I see them crashing onto the shore. They must make a sound."

I was building a sand castle. The thick sand walls were water-dampened and -hardened. Three tall mud-dripped turrets stood atop a fantastic-looking structure adorned with battlements and scooped window openings. A bridge crossed a moat. And I was now sculpting small sand soldiers to guard the whole affair. I had no time to tell my father what things sounded like. I pretended I didn't see his hands.

He shook me, not too gently. "What do the waves sound like?" he repeated.

It was no use. *Here we go again*, I thought. "Loud," I answered him without thinking. "Loud they must be," he signed patiently, "but many things are loud. I feel loudness through the soles of my feet. But every loud thing must be loud in its own way." He had me there.

"Well," I sighed while signing, my shoulders lifting to signal that I was thinking, my features arranging themselves in an expression suggesting that I was not sure of my answer but would do the best I could.

"They sound *wet* when they crash down on the sand."

As soon as I said that, I knew my father would ask what *wet* sounded like. No sooner had my fingers touched my lips, and then opened and closed against my thumbs as they made the sign for *wet*, than my father demanded, "What kind of wet? Wet like a wild river? Wet like soft rain? Wet like sad tears?"

I was stumped. "Wet like waves!" was all I could come up with at first. I finally signed, "Waves sound like a billion wet drops breaking apart when they smack down on the hard sand, all the tiny sounds joining to make one great sound. A *wet* falling ocean sound," I added desperately.

My father took me into his arms and held me. Letting go, he got down on his knees in the sand and signed, "That's better. I understand now."

Just then Mort shook my father's shoulders. "Lou! Lou! Look! Here comes Sally."

Sure enough, my mother had entered the deaf circle, holding my brother's hand. She was in her blue two-piece knitted-wool bathing suit. She wore a white rubber bathing cap with tiny yellow rubber flowers attached, covering her close-cropped black hair. She always wore her hair short in the summer. She looked beautiful. Before my mother even set down her beach chair, Ben was in her face, signing wildly like a windmill in a windstorm.

I could swear I saw my father mutter to himself in sign, "I'll murder that guy."

My mother signed a greeting to Ben, then held his arms to his sides, silencing him, and turned to my father with a smile from ear to ear.

If my father had been an Eskimo Pie, he would have melted in the warmth of that smile.

12

The Triangle and the Chihuahua

Long ago, children in Brooklyn public schools were exposed to more than academic and "practical" subjects. In addition to art appreciation, there was music appreciation. But this form of appreciation found me as wanting as art appreciation did, since I was virtually tone deaf.

In my very first music class our teacher had us sing "God Bless America," while she tinkled away on her slightly off-key piano. As early fall sunlight streamed through the tall grimy windows of the music appreciation room, slanting dusty bars of golden light illuminated our efforts to mouth the lyrics. Unfortunately for me, one of those revealing bars of light illuminated my lips, which had remained closed throughout the duration of the song. My failure to participate did not go unnoticed.

"Myron," the teacher inquired, "has the cat got your tongue?"

"No, ma'am," I managed to get out.

"Let's do it over," she said to the class, "so Myron can join in."

I tried, I surely did, but after only a few bars the piano died, and with it my public school singing career.

"Myron," the teacher said ever so gently, "from now on you will be in charge of the most important element in the overall success of our chorus."

And with that she placed in my hands a piece of metal in the shape of a triangle.

"What's this?" I asked. "It looks like a triangle."

"*Exactly,*" she exclaimed. "How clever of you to understand so quickly."

From that moment on I was never to sing a single note. Instead I stood at the rear of the chorus, holding my triangle by a string grasped in one hand while striking it gently, pretty much as the mood struck me, with a slim metal wand held in the other. Of course, the occasional slight tinkles of sound were drowned out by the robust voices of my classmates.

"Practice," my teacher instructed me after presenting me with the triangle. "Practice makes perfect," she added, and sent me home with the triangle without another word. *To do what?* I wondered. *To practice,* I surmised.

And so it was that I proudly climbed the three flights of stairs that afternoon, triangle held carefully under my arm, steel wand safely in my pocket. Greeting my mother and brother at the door to our apartment, I waved the triangle at them, very full of myself.

"I'm a musician," I signed to her, while also announcing it out loud to my brother. "My teacher said I'm the most important part of our chorus."

"That's nice," my mother, a daughter of the Great Depression, signed right back. "Sit. You look hungry. I'll make you both some matzoh brei."

"But I have to practice. My teacher said so."

"Eat first—you'll have more strength to practice," she signed emphatically, her hands moving away from her chest, turning into fists.

My mother always said that her theory about life was that any problem could be faced, and overcome, with nothing more than a full stomach.

That evening, as usual, my father came home with the day's newspaper under his arm.

"There is much to talk about," he signed dramatically to my brother and me. "The news today is exciting."

After dinner every evening, while my mother was doing the dishes, my father, brother, and I sat at the kitchen table while he signed the headlines to us. Then he explained the importance of each headline. Most of the news was about the happenings in Europe and England and about two funny men, one short and fat with a thrust-out jaw, the other with a bad haircut and a spot of mustache on his upper lip. My father could imitate Hitler as well as Charlie Chaplin. Although the news in Europe was bad, my father had me and my brother laughing while he mimed Mussolini's strutting walk and Hitler's silly salute and his promise to take over the whole world. Little did we know just how close he would come.

Mussolini and Hitler were the bad guys. FDR was the good guy, with Winnie Churchill a close second. Things were very clear to me in those days.

"I have something exciting to tell you, too," my signs interrupted my father. "I'm the backbone of the class chorus," I added in finger-spelling, as I had no sign for *backbone*.

I ran to my room and quickly returned with my triangle.

"See," I signed. "This is a triangle, and my teacher is counting on me to learn how to use it. 'Practice,' she said, 'and the chorus will follow you.'"

"My son, the musician," my father signed in all seriousness. "How would you like to have a chihuahua?" He spelled with exquisite care and exactitude. Watching his fingers spell this new long word filled with so many *h*'s connected with so many *u*'s and assorted *a*'s left me dizzy. And right in the middle of an *h* and a *u*, his face broke into a broad grin. I was well aware of my father's sense of humor and how he would often set me up for one of his jokes. But I figured I'd play the straight man and go along with him on this one, like George Burns always did with Gracie on the radio.

"What is a chihuahua?" I finger-spelled right back to him, adding a dozen extra *h*'s, *u*'s, and *a*'s.

"It's a dog," he signed, patting his knee and snapping his fingers. Then so he was perfectly clear, his open right hand, imitating a paw, brushed his right ear repeatedly. "A very little dog, with very big ears."

Since we lived in Brooklyn, in a small apartment, the subject of dogs of any size rarely if ever came up as a topic of conversation. But as I watched my father's signs, I could actually see this tiny, alert dog with its inquisitive, intelligent face. My father's signs were so expressive, I could almost hear the squeaky bark emanating from this sketch of a dog that he painted on the air.

"Xavier Cugat," he finger-spelled the name, "the great rumba bandleader, has a chihuahua in his pocket when he leads his band. And now that you have a triangle, I think you could use a dog in your pocket as well."

And with that he gently pulled my mother from the sink, apron and all, and began to twirl her around the kitchen, the two of them smoothly sliding across the waxed linoleum floor to a rumba beat that only they could hear.

The night of the school concert finally arrived. The auditorium was filled to capacity. Not a single Brooklyn parent was about to miss hearing their precious, incredibly gifted child perform that special evening.

My father, mother, and brother came early so that they would have front-row seats. Although they wouldn't be able to hear me banging on my triangle, my father and mother wanted to be close enough to see me and imagine the beautiful sounds I must surely be making.

Noticing my parents talking to each other in exaggerated signs, my teacher moved me to the front of the chorus, to the very edge of the stage.

With the passing of so many years, my memory of that evening is dim. I do vaguely recall my futile attempts to strike my triangle in time with the music, but I was always chasing the rhythm, always a few beats behind.

Yet my memory is crystal clear when it comes to the look of undisguised pride on my father's and mother's faces, as they sat enraptured—there is no other word for it—by my musicality. Being stone deaf, they heard not a sound, and I, forlornly beating away at my triangle, was deaf in my own way.

*A*fter the concert I continued to hold on to the image that my father's hands had painted of Xavier Cugat's chihuahua, peeking out of the bandleader's pocket at the dancers box-stepping the rumba. My father was the artist of that picture, and like so many others that he had created for me, it now hung with the rest of them in the picture gallery of my mind. So sharp was that image that I now wanted the dog that he had sketched with such vividness.

The best way to begin my campaign for a dog, I reasoned, was with my mother. She would be the one member of the family who would be around to care for my dog when my brother and I were at school and my father was at work. I needed her approval before I approached my father.

I planned my campaign well and with exacting care, taking into account all that I knew about my mother. Surely, I reasoned, I would *not* bring up the subject on an empty stomach. Only after eating my fill, preferably to near bursting, would I talk about a dog to my mother, for only then could I be sure of being able to talk without being interrupted by the dreaded command, "Sit. Eat."

But when I did finally raise the subject, without hesitation my mother launched into a long rambling story about the time when she was a child and had also wanted a dog. Her reasons were quite different from my own.

"Every Sunday night my father took me by subway from my home in Coney Island to my school, the Lexington School for the Deaf, on Lexington Avenue in the city.

"I attended classes all week long and slept in the dorm with my friends at night. That was where we learned sign language—first from the older girls, and then from one another. We talked in sign all night long, since signing was absolutely forbidden by our hearing teachers during the daytime. Oh, we were so naughty." Here she made the sign for *bad*, but the gestures that accompanied it, lips compressed into a sly grin and shoulders lifted in a girls-will-be-girls shrug, signaled that what she meant was: not really *bad* but rather *naughty*.

By now, my proficiency in sign had grown to the point that I was able without even thinking to discern the subtleties of my parents' language. A sign could have multiple meanings, depending upon the context and the manner in which it was conveyed: the shape of the hands in making the sign, the utilization of facial grammar, the positioning of the hands relative to the body, and indeed the use of the entire body. Thus *bad* became *naughty* that day, but with my mother's expressive ability in sign, it might just as well have become *evil, nasty,* or *wicked,* depending on the context. Through my parents' hands, bodies, and faces, individual signs recombined effortlessly to communicate volumes of information.

I always marveled at my mother's signing ability and was aware that it was more fluid, expressive, and expansive than my father's. I had always assumed that that was because my mother went to deaf school at a younger age than my father did, and so learned the language earlier. But underlying that was the difference in their basic personalities. My father was practical, direct, forceful, and narrowly focused—and so was his signing. My mother, on the other hand, was more emotional and very much a dreamer, as well as a born storyteller. I could get lost in her picturesque, all-enveloping signs.

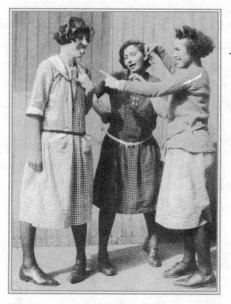

My mother and her friends signing to one another at the Lexington School for the Deaf, circa 1922.

"When the lights were turned out," she continued, "we went to the bathroom, where a light was always on, and we talked till our eyes refused to stay open. We loved to talk to one another in our language. We lived for sign, and the ability to communicate with one another was like the water of life, our oasis of language and meaning, in the midst of the huge expanse of desert silence and incomprehension that was the greater hearing world.

"Every Friday night my father came to get me, and together we took the subway back to Brooklyn. We had to take two different subway lines to get to Coney Island, the end of the Sea Beach line. The trip seemed to take forever, and in all that time my father said not a word to me. He did not know a single sign, other than the few he had made up during the years I was a child. These were feeble signs that I was embarrassed to repeat to my school friends. They were primitive crude things lacking grace and meaning. They made me feel simpleminded, almost backward, and they embarrassed me even when I used them with my father and mother. That was the speech of an idiot. I was not an idiot."

My mother's hands stopped in midsentence. Suspended in the air in front of her body, they seemed to be thinking. Remembering.

"I loved my mother. I loved my father. I loved my younger sister and my three younger brothers. But not one of them knew me. They never learned my language. We were strangers all the years of my childhood. There were times I wished I was blind, not deaf. Then I could have heard my mother's voice. I could have told her my fears and wishes, and my love for her."

My mother had never talked to me this way before. I began to be sorry I had asked for a dog. I did not understand why my request had triggered these memories, but I felt I had been selfish. And somewhere deep down I felt angry. I was angry that my mother had suffered so. I felt a sense of helplessness for the first time in my life, mirroring what my mother must have felt growing up. I felt the unfairness of her situation. My father was a fighter, a battler against the daily cruelties that the hearing unthinkingly levied against him. But my mother was cut from a different cloth; she wore the cloak of resignation. She was vulnerable. As I grappled with these conflicting emotions, she continued her story.

"When my father and I arrived at our apartment in Coney Island on Friday night, my mother would greet me at the door with a tight smile on her thin lips, but always with a hug and a special light in her eyes.

"She immediately took my hand and led me to the kitchen, which smelled of onions and garlic and Shabbes chicken.

"This was my mother's language of love: her cooking. Stingy with her emotions, never really smiling, she expressed her feelings for me in the thousand meals she prepared for me alone, often feeding me by hand long after I was old enough to feed myself."

My mother's signs made my mouth water, and my eyes filled with tears. I was both sad and hungry watching my mother's story unfold through her expressive hands.

"After eating, I went to my room, where I stayed pretty much the entire weekend. My mother tried shooing me out the door, her crude signs suggesting I go downstairs and play with the other children. But I wouldn't go. When I was younger, I tried to play with the other kids in the street. But they would run away from me in different directions, meeting later at some prearranged place, like an alleyway, where they regrouped, giggling at how they had escaped."

She stopped moving her hands and smiled at me.

"But I was going to tell you my story about a dog, not all this stuff about chickens," and she laughed.

"I was a lonely child, always lonely in my own home. I could talk to no one in my family, and no one learned to talk to me. I wanted a dog to keep me company. One day I asked my father for a dog for my next birthday. He, perhaps out of guilt, readily agreed; he never denied me anything, except himself. For without a language to share, I never knew him.

"One Saturday morning, while in a half sleep, I felt a furry busyness and a wet, hot tongue against my cheek. Awakening, I saw pressed against my face a bundle of orange fur. It was a puppy. I held the squirming orange fur ball at arm's length, turning him this way and that, while he struggled to get free. He was perfect, and he was mine.

"I said thank you . . . thank you . . . thank you . . . to my father, but as usual, when I spoke, his face squeezed shut. My parents always winced at the sound of my voice, so I knew it must be ugly. But for once I didn't care. I had a dog of my own.

"I named him Chubby. He would follow me wherever I went, from room to room, up and down the stairs of our apartment building, in and out of bed, everywhere. He loved me, and I loved him more than I had ever loved anything in my life.

"And he grew. Boy, did he grow. Later I found out he was a full-blooded chow. They grow very large, and their full orange coat makes them seem even bigger.

"Chubby was strong, and he loved the snow. In the winter he would grasp the collar of my little brother's coat in his mouth and would pull him on the seat of his pants through the snow, and over the ice, up and down our block.

"Chubby and I had our own language. We understood each other perfectly. He understood me when I spoke a command. And not once did he wince or turn away at the sound of my voice. I had merely to whisper his name from another room, and he would come bounding down the hallway to my side. And I taught him signs. Chubby learned sign, whereas my parents and brothers and sister never did. I began to think Chubby was a lot smarter than all of them.

"Now my weekends at home went by in a blur of orange fur, and I wasn't lonely for one second of the time. It was hard to say goodbye to Chubby every Monday morning, when my father took me back to my school. But he was always there, anticipating my arrival, every Friday night when I returned."

I did not recall my mother ever looking as happy as she did when she recounted what she remembered of her dog from so long ago, her childhood friend.

"But one day I lost Chubby forever. He had been jumping on a neighbor's boy, who had been teasing him. When I went to pull him off, he bit me. I know he didn't know it was me. He was just reacting like any dog would—he was protecting himself. But his bite was deep, and I was rushed to Coney Island Hospital, where the wound on my hand was stitched closed.

"When my father brought me home from the hospital, Chubby was waiting for me by the door as usual. He looked sad. I forgave him.

"The next weekend Chubby was gone. I found out later that my father had sold him to the iceman for five dollars. I never had a dog again."

Suddenly I didn't want a dog anymore. I had a hundred friends. I was never lonely. I had too much to do to take care of a silly old dog.

"What's to eat?" I asked my mother. "I'm hungry."

This, of course, was music that even my mother's deaf ears could hear.

There was no talk of a dog ever again.

13
My Father's Language

*T*here is a wall in my home that displays a score of old family photos. But no physical photograph is as sharp as the mental picture I have of my father. In memory I see my father with his surprisingly small, slender nose, thick black hair parted just off the precise middle of his head with razor sharpness, and eyes like a pair of dark reflecting pools framed by questioning eyebrows, through which he saw a world that he struggled, often with limited success, to decode. His mouth is small and empty. It contains no language. His lips are thin. They shape no words. My father's language is in his hands.

My father's hands were strong. His language was strong. He did not try to become invisible by making small signs in public. His signs were not furtive, fearful, timid, or apologetic. On the silvered screen of memory the snapshot images are transformed into a movie, and signs are flung powerfully from his hands like wild birds taking flight. And like the beating of a wild bird's wings, my father's hands would not be contained. "Look at me, world," they pronounced. "I'm a deaf man. I'm proud. Hearing people can go to hell, I don't care."

When he was angry, his signs were angry. His face expressed anger. And anger flowed from his body until you could feel its heat. My father's anger was mainly directed at the hearing world. Although he had long since accepted the unthinking hostility that hearing people directed at him on a daily basis—they were ignorant of deaf ways, he reasoned—what did set him off was their indifference. They seemed to ignore him, as if he, a deaf man, were simply invisible to them.

When my father was happy, his signs were light and fanciful, and they soared. His happiness registered in his face, and his entire body expanded in joy.

Above all things, his family brought him happiness. His signs embraced us.

One night as we were sitting at the kitchen table after dinner, my father told my brother and me:

"Hearing people talk only with the mouth. Hearing words tumble from the mouth, one word after another word, like a long word train. The meaning is not clear until the caboose word comes out of the mouth tunnel. These are only dry words, like dead insects. Mouth-talk is like a painting with no color. You can see shape. Understand an idea. But it's flat, like a black and white picture. There is no life in a black and white picture.

"My language is not a black and white language. The language of my hands and face and body is a Technicolor language. When I am angry, my language is red-hot like the sun. When I am happy, my language is blue like the ocean, and green like a meadow, and yellow like pretty flowers.

"My language is God's language. He put His language in my hands for all my time on earth. In heaven I will have no need for sign. I will talk directly to God."

My father had made himself a student of how spoken language compares to sign language. Now he decided it was time to give my brother and me a demonstration of the difference between the two.

"Now you mouth-talk," he signed. "Say *drum*."

He watched my mouth carefully as I said, "Drum."

"Say *thunder*."

He put his open palm in front of my mouth as I said, "Thunder."

"Say *crash*."

I said, "Crash."

"I cannot see a loud sound when you say these hearing mouth-words," my father signed. "And I do not feel a loud sound coming from your mouth."

"Yes," I answered him. "To make my words explain how loud a drum sounds, or how loud the thunder is, or how loud the crash is, I have to use other words, words that describe the original word. Adjectives."

"I know hearing adjective words," he answered with derision. "Adjectives are decoration words, like silver tinsel on a green Christmas tree. They are not real words with their own meaning. A beautiful green tree needs no decoration. Such a tree is most beautiful in the ground and not in a living room with its beauty covered up with tinsel, lights, and hanging balls. Your mouth-talk is a weak thing. It needs many more words to explain the original word."

He thought a minute. "Watch me now talk with my hands."

My father signed *drum*. His hands held invisible drumsticks, and he slowly began to beat an invisible drum. Softly.

My brother and I sat mesmerized at the sight of our father's closed hands rising and falling.

Then his hands moved faster, more forcefully, and I saw the ends of the drumsticks striking the skin of the drumhead and began to "hear" his hands, while Irwin laughed with glee.

Suddenly a look of intense concentration spread across my

father's face, and his shoulders and body bent into the beating of his hands as they banged away with the now-visible drumsticks on the now-visible drum. I listened to the sound of his face and body and hands, all indivisible, and the sound was deafening. I covered my ears, and my brother followed my lead and covered his as well.

My father stopped banging. His hands were empty. The drumsticks had disappeared. The drum had disappeared. The sound had disappeared.

"My language is a picture language," he signed, breathing heavily. "There is no need to explain."

His point made, my father smiled and picked up the newspaper that he had brought home from work that day.

"Come watch," my father said. "Now I make magic. I will make for you and Irwin four-cornered newspaper hats. Hats like my pals and me wear in the newspaper plant to keep the ink mist off our heads."

As my mother dried the last of the dishes, my father carefully spread the paper out on the kitchen table. Selecting a perfect section, one that had been mechanically folded exactly down the center, his hands began to create magic. Folding the double-spread first this way and that, while scoring the edges with his strong nails, he tucked and folded the sheet of newsprint until, out of all the folds and creases, the shape of a hat emerged.

Tucking the final folds into place, he opened the shaped newsprint, and suddenly, before my eyes, he held a three-dimensional newspaper hat where but moments earlier there had been a one-dimensional sheet of paper. He gently placed it on my head. Somehow, miraculously, the hat was—as it always was—a perfect fit.

"You're a printer now. Like me. No ink will get in your hair to make your pillow dirty and make Mother Sarah angry."

He then repeated the process and placed a small newspaper hat on my brother's head. We wore our newspaper hats to bed.

I often dreamed I was a printer, standing on the printing press floor alongside my father. He wore a newspaper hat. There was no ink in his hair.

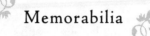

Memorabilia

The Palmer Method

I came home from school one day, my notebook filled with lines of gorgeous letters all in a row, bounding across the page like a herd of prancing gazelles. Sandwiched between these lines of soaring grace were leaden lines of crawling caterpillars.

This had been my first exposure to the dreaded Palmer Method of penmanship, which the school authorities of Brooklyn, in their wisdom, had determined was essential to the education of every budding street scholar. In my particular case, it was deemed critical. "Myron, what on earth are these words?" my teacher had said, at her wit's end. "This page looks like the yard of a chicken run. What could these chicken tracks possibly mean?" I tried to explain, but in truth, some of the words were indecipherable even to me; this was impressive, as I had written them just a moment before.

As I listened to my traitorous classmates laughing, I watched in awe as my teacher proceeded to fill my notebook with lines of graceful, elegant letters—in alternating capitals and lower case.

"Now, Myron, take your notebook home and *practice!*"

That evening, after my mother had cleared the supper dishes from the kitchen table, I practiced my penmanship. In the blank lines between my teacher's beautiful gazelle-like words, I scrawled my ugly, clumsy counterparts, as my father sat across from me, reading his paper.

Setting the newspaper aside, my father turned my notebook around so that he could look at what I had written.

"What in heaven's name are you doing?" he signed. The look on his face was one of pure puzzlement.

"I'm practicing my penmanship."

"Is *that* what it is?" my father said skeptically. "So why can't I read it?" he added—unnecessarily, I thought.

Not meaning to be rude but realizing this line of conversation was not leading anywhere that I wanted to go, I took the notebook back and resumed my tortured, crabbed, and—even to my mind—pathetic squiggles across the page.

Line after line of miserable . . . what? Yes, I realized, they were exactly as my teacher had said: chicken tracks.

I laid down my pen in utter frustration. I was a beaten kid. And besides, my hand hurt.

Looking up at my father, I saw him break into the most exaggerated signs, punctuated with carefully sculpted finger-spelled letters of the alphabet. It was as if he were cutting those letters from a block of marble one by one, each letter perfect.

His signs looped and soared with the ornamental elegance of a peacock, blended with the agility of a long-tailed swallow.

"That's *my* Palmer Method," he signed, picking up his newspaper again.

14

Parent-Teacher Night

$\mathcal{T}$ he year I turned nine, I was faced with my ultimate challenge as intermediary between my father and the outside world: the dreaded Parent-Teacher Night.

When I learned that our parents were invited—and attendance was definitely not optional—to a conference with our teachers regarding our progress (or lack of it in my case) in our schoolwork and our social development (*Deportment? Works and plays well with others? Conduct? Good grief!*), this news chilled me to the bone. I was sure that my father would insist that I accompany them to the event. For something this important I knew he would not be content merely to shuffle cryptic, tediously scrawled notes back and forth with my impatient teacher. He would want me to act—as I had since I was six—as his interpreter, so that he could have access to the same full understanding of the exchange between teacher and parent that any hearing person would unthinkingly enjoy.

Holding on to some small fragment of hope that I could get out of going, I explained to my father that we, the children, were not invited. But my father insisted on my presence, as he always did on any occasion of note that required him to interact with the hearing world.

This occasion, of course, was different from any of the others. Up until now I had been merely a glass window through which language passed from the hearing to my deaf father, and then in the other direction—I was the facilitator. But now I would be the subject, the whole point of the exercise that evening. The thoughts and opinions I would be passing on to my father and teacher, in sign and spoken language, would consist of highly subjective opinions about myself. I was horrified. Only seven short days separated me from the upcoming ordeal. I passed over and through the intervening hours as if I were being dragged over hot coals.

My concerns were manifold and complex. Up until now my entire world, the world I inhabited with my deaf mother and father, had been my Brooklyn block—actually only half of it, as I rarely if ever ventured past the midway point. In this world I was known as the hearing son of two deaf parents, no more, no less—and best of all, no big deal.

When my mother called my name, *Mhhhaaarinnn,* from our third-floor apartment window in her sharp deaf voice, no one even turned his or her head to see where that keening sound came from. When my father cheered me on during games of stickball and touch football in his hard harsh voice, my friends barely noticed. And when my father signed to me, and I signed back, no one stared. The rhythmic movements of our arms and hands and bodies as we signed were as natural as the waving of the branches of the few trees on our block in the occasional breeze from Coney Island.

On this block, in this world, I was unremarkable.

But now all that would change. Now, in a few painfully short days, I would be with my parents in a huge auditorium filled with teachers and parents—strangers who had never encountered a deaf person, or heard a deaf voice, or seen what to them would appear a meaningless, almost demented, arm-waving, grimacing, squeaking, and scowling performance.

Moreover, I would have to endure my father's request that I translate into spoken words his admiration of my numerous skills and attributes, each and every one of them, to my teacher.

In turn, I would have to interpret my teacher's honest, critical, but oh-so-constructive opinions of my shortcomings, also one by one.

The evening inevitably arrived, on schedule.

"Myron, please tell your parents I'm very happy to finally meet them," my teacher said in her pleasantly soft-pitched voice.

I smiled and interpreted word for word, my facial grammar expressing her happiness.

"Myron, please tell the teacher that we are as well," signed and voiced my father, in exaggerated sign and harsh voice.

I cringed and interpreted word for word.

"Myron, please tell your parents that although you are a good student, you are a severe discipline problem."

"The teacher says I'm a pleasure to have in her class."

"Tell them that if you don't improve in deportment, conduct, and paying attention, I'll have to recommend that you be left back a grade."

"My teacher says that at the rate I'm learning, she may recommend me for skipping a grade," I signed creatively.

"Furthermore," my teacher said in her sweetly modulated voice, "tell your parents that you are the worst discipline problem I've ever encountered in all of my twenty-two years of teaching in Brooklyn schools. Myron, you are truly unique."

"My teacher says that she sees a bright future for me, perhaps as a surgeon or an airline pilot."

By now my mother was beaming.

But my father, who had watched the very active and prolonged movement of my teacher's lips throughout the entire exchange, was scowling with marked skepticism.

"Bullshit!" he signed to me in our home sign for the word. "*Bullshit*," he repeated in exasperation.

"Now, by God, tell me exactly what the teacher is saying," he signed in his no-nonsense sign. My father, who could read the face of a hearing person as an Egyptologist can read the Rosetta Stone, had cracked the hieroglyphics of my teacher's face and gestures. He knew the gist of what she was saying, and now he wanted the details. The jig was up. Now I was back to performing my disappearing act—in an instant I became the clear glass through which the unedited thoughts and comments of my teacher and my father would pass, back and forth.

Looking at my father's grim face and angry gestures, my teacher said in the voice she reserved for speaking to me when I disobeyed her request to be quiet in class, "Myron, what have you been telling your father?"

"Well . . ." I began, but couldn't continue.

"Myron, tell your father *exactly* what I'm saying to him now."

I visibly cringed.

Seeing my discomfort, my dear teacher took pity on me.

"Myron is a good boy. He reads well and is obviously intelligent, but he has a discipline problem." Then she smiled and said, "He has ants in his pants." Reflecting on her own metaphor, she added, "And there are times I'm tempted to *squash* him, like an ant."

The sign for *ant* is iconic and graphic: the closed left hand is the body of an ant and sits above the back of the right hand, which moves forward while the fingers wiggle furiously like an ant's legs. In my newfound honesty, to eliminate any doubt in my father's mind as to *exactly* what my teacher meant by this statement, I followed with the second version of this sign: the hands are closed in fists, and the right extended thumbnail comes down repeatedly against the left thumbnail, squashing an army of ants between the thumbnails. I executed this last sign with such descriptive power that my mother smiled—and nodded vigorously in agreement—while my father collapsed in convulsive laughter that was interrupted by an emphatically barked "YES! YES!" followed by his sign for "Sometimes, same me! Squash Myron like an ant."

As my father made the exaggerated signs for *squash Myron like an ant,* my teacher joined in the hilarity, all at my expense. But I didn't care. I had escaped any further elaboration of my transgressions in her class.

Soon, however, I noticed that this lively exchange had made our little group the center of attention for every parent and teacher in the room. I saw the stares and gaping mouths and looks of astonishment on their faces.

Piss off, I thought. *I'll be as tough as my father.* And I proceeded to stare right back at them.

That night after we returned to our apartment and my father paid the neighbor's child who had watched Irwin while we were out, my mother made hot cocoa for Irwin and me. She topped it off with my favorite—fresh whipped cream that she made by hand with an egg beater in a cold metal bowl. When I finished drinking my cocoa, she let me scoop the remaining fluffy pile of whipped cream from the bowl directly into my mouth—and when my brother complained, into his mouth as well. This was a rare treat for Irwin, as she thought the habit quite unsanitary, and she was always very protective of him. I couldn't imagine why, but my mother seemed pleased with me.

My father was another matter. He was as serious as I had ever seen him be with me. Looking at me sternly, he said, "Myron, no more of your foolishness in school. I expect a better report from your teacher at the next parent-teacher meeting." Then, while holding my gaze, he hesitated and added, "And if you don't . . . ," and he made the sign for squashing an ant—and burst into laughter.

Memorabilia

The Spider-Man of Ninth Street

T wenty years before the nerdy high school nonentity Peter Parker was bitten on his hand by a radioactive spider, transforming him instantly into Spider-Man, I decided I could climb up the brick face of my apartment house wall. I arrived at this startling conclusion after only a little practice and even less thought.

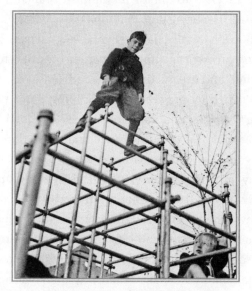

I'm practicing to be Spider-Man.

Like every other kid in Brooklyn in 1943, I was a great fan of the King of the Jungle, Tarzan. I saw every one of his movies at our local movie house, the Avalon Theater, the week it was released. And I bought every one of his comic books the minute it hit the rack at our local candy store. Indeed, although I wasn't much of a student in my school-based subjects, I was a summa cum laude in anything depicted in movies and comic books. Tarzan's extraordinary ability to climb trees like an ape, and to swing from trees on the vines that grew in their upper reaches, inspired me to attempt my own vine-swinging feats. Thus I swiped a length of clothesline and fashioned a Brooklyn version of an African vine.

One day, with my "vine" wound tightly around my waist, I climbed a tree that stood in our backyard. All day long I scampered up and down the length of that tree, my clothesline vine attached to one of its topmost branches so that I could swing in soaring arcs that took me over our neighbor's garage roof. Eventually, having exhausted the possibilities of simulating an African jungle experience in one tree, I lay along a limb and dreamed of further adventures.

Emboldened by my success at climbing a tree trunk and swinging from the end of a clothesline, I decided that, like Tarzan, I would use this means of transportation to move about my "jungle"—West Ninth Street, Brooklyn, New York.

But my "jungle" was rather sparse, its trees few and far between. Swinging from one to another required skills that would have taxed even Cheetah, not to mention Tarzan. Still, I was determined to expand my fantasy to its outermost limits, and so I soon settled on an interesting alternative: the telephone cables that snaked their way, high overhead, from pole to pole, down the backyards of my street. Looking up at them with my hyperactive ten-year-old imagination, I could easily visualize them as the thick jungle canopy I would soon be negotiating with my clothesline.

One afternoon, my "vine" wound tightly around my waist, where it performed no function except in my mind, I climbed a telephone pole in my backyard. Grasping the cable at the top, I began my progress above the backyards of my block, making my way slowly, hand over hand, from one pole to the next, until I reached Avenue P, the end of my street. Not bad, I thought, then reversed my position on the cable and made my way in the opposite direction until I reached Quentin Road. Had Tarzan as a boy lived in Brooklyn, could he have done any better?

If any neighbors had happened to glance out their rear windows, they would have seen a kid with a clothesline wound in coils around his waist, dangling from the telephone wires, with a determined expression of absolute concentration on his face. Yes, I *was* the king of my jungle. Fortunately, no one saw me—or reported me to my parents, as they would certainly have done if they had—and I was able to perform this feat several days in a row until, tiring of the rather restricted movements available to me on the single telephone line running up and down the "rooftop" of my jungle, I returned to my ample collection of Tarzan comic books to investigate possibilities for further adventures.

Using the amazing powers of deduction with which all Brooklyn kids were genetically endowed to enable them to transform their environment into something more exotic, I hit on the idea that the brick face of my apartment house was the sheer face of a jungle escarpment. Of course, I didn't know what an escarpment was, but when I looked upward at the wall, indelibly etched in my mind was the image of

Tarzan climbing a sheer cliff face, followed closely by a lion. Holding that image in my mind, I imagined a lion on West Ninth Street stealthily stalking me.

And so it was that one day I found myself clinging to the face of my apartment house wall, like a spider on steroids, fingers and sneaker-toes embedded between the bricks, two stories above the ground. It was slow going, but brick by brick I proceeded upward, the hot breath of the lion warming my feet, its deep cough throbbing in my ear.

Ignoring the real-life screams of the neighborhood mothers rising from the street below me, I crawled up and up, mindful of the fire escape railings just inches to my right. My fail-safe plan was to grab the rail of a handy fire escape if I should begin to fall.

Just at the moment I was sure I had escaped the lion, Mrs. Abromovitz emerged from her bedroom window, rags in hand, to perform her once-a-week window-cleaning ritual. Settling her ample rump comfortably on the windowsill, she lowered the overhead window onto her lap for security, turned, and saw me clinging to the wall, inches from her face. Her single scream put to shame the collective yells from the gaggle of neighborhood *yentas* below. Theirs were but a murmuring breeze, split by the thunder of her voice.

The lowered window kept her nailed to the windowsill, as she sat stunned in fright.

I froze, stuck to the face of the building, paralyzed by the sound. Regaining my wits, I knew I had to get out of there quickly. But up or down? Down below waited my imaginary foul-breathed lion and the outraged *yentas*—infinitely more fearsome predators—so up I went, up to our apartment's third-floor fire escape.

As my mother was deaf, she did not hear me climb through her bedroom window. And since I had my own key to our apartment, she did not know that I had entered it from the fire escape. Not for the first time I realized that for a kid like me, having deaf parents had some practical advantages.

But I knew there would be a reckoning.

That evening, when my father came home from work, three of our neighbors were stationed at our front door. They had all written down their fervid accounts of my escapade, and now they jabbed the resulting narratives in my father's weary face.

Mrs. Abromovitz had yet to emerge from her apartment. Her meek husband was faithfully attending to her as she lay in her bed, to which she had immediately retired upon regaining her senses.

My father and I had a most interesting conversation that evening, a conversation that taxed to the utmost my signing comprehension. But, as ever, my father's expressive use of his beloved language left no doubt in my mind what lay in store for me should I *ever again* attempt a similar stunt.

The lion was not seen or heard from again on our block. The fearsome sounds of those *yentas* no doubt drove him back to Africa.

15

A Boy in Uniform

Every night after dinner, while my mother was doing the evening dishes, my father sat at the kitchen table with my brother and me and read to us—in sign—from the first page of the *New York Daily News*, which his labors in the composing room had helped to create. In its early years World War II was going badly. We were losing on every front, one battle after another. "Don't worry," his hands told Irwin and me with perfect conviction, "America has never lost a war."

I could read most of the words on the front page for myself. Even the ones I didn't know, I could sound out. But I much preferred that my father read the front page to me. Words like *war*, and *battles*, and *army*, and *shell*, and *bomb* were just words to me, as were *wounded* and *dead*. But when my father's expressive hands turned these words into sign, they came alive. In the movement of his hands, I could see the fall of bombs, the flight of shells, and the movements of vast armies; I could hear the cries of the wounded and the stillness of death. His hands told me of the Bataan Death March, and I could see our weary soldiers dragging their broken bodies along the endless dusty roads, and I could feel the jabs of bayonet points as their cruel Japanese guards prodded them. I could see the shells erupting on the decks of battleships at the Battle of Midway, the fires and explosions bursting into the air, the sailors abandoning ship as jagged holes appeared at the waterline, and the oil-stained sea becoming clotted with sailors clinging to floating debris. My brother would sit at his side of the table, too young to comprehend what all the excitement was about, but fascinated by the dramatic signs and thrilled by every minute of the performance.

I had a vivid imagination as a young boy and could readily turn words into images in my mind. But the constant commerce between words and signs that was so much a part of my life greatly expanded this ability.

The evening readings with my father were the high point of my day, and I became a great student of the war. My friends would have to wait for the Pathé newsreel that was shown every Saturday afternoon on the silver screen at our local movie house for a visual chronicle of the progress of the war. I, on the other hand, could watch it every night of the week on the human screen of my father's hands.

In 1944 the tide of war was turning in our favor. We were on the march. I thrilled to my father's signs every night, as he read to me the headlines that trumpeted the advances our soldiers were making up the boot of Italy.

In June Rome was liberated.

That same month the Allies landed on the beaches of Normandy. D-Day had finally arrived. Slowly but surely our troops were slogging their way to Paris.

The newspaper was filled with pictures of soldiers in uniform; soldiers in foxholes; soldiers in chow lines; soldiers at the front; and even dead soldiers. All wore uniforms of one kind or another, theirs and ours.

I wanted a uniform of my own.

My mother's youngest brother, Milton, was a captain in the army, a paratrooper posted somewhere in Europe, and then in Burma. He sent me a bayonet holder and a bandolier. I wore them around the apartment.

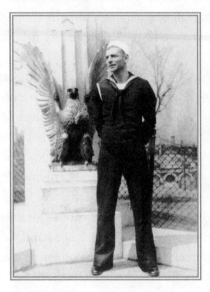

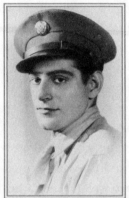

Harry (left) and my mother's youngest brother, Milton (above)

Harry, another of my mother's brothers, was a sailor on a battleship somewhere in the Pacific Ocean. He sent me a sailor's hat. It was spanking white and broken in quite nicely, with creases in all the right places, and I liked to wear it tilted over one eye at a rakish angle. With my sailor hat on my head, I marched around our apartment, walking splayfooted as I imagined my uncle did when manning the deck at the height of a storm in the Pacific, the waves crashing over the bow, roller upon roller.

Our apartment was small. I was constantly underfoot. And as my mother liked to wash and wax the kitchen floor every day—hourly, it seemed to me—she often chased me out of the apartment and into our third-floor hallway. My brother, however, had to remain inside with her, ever close, where she could keep an eye on him.

Soon the older kids in the building, all wearing scraps of a uniform—an odd hat here, a cracked leather belt there—joined me. We stomped up and down the marble-floored hallways and clattered up and down the metal stairways, singing:

"You're in the Army now. You're not behind the plow. You'll never get rich by digging a ditch. You're in the Army now."

Our combined voices echoed through the halls and up and down the stairwells, until angry neighbors flung open the door of every apartment and shouted at us to *shut up!*, threatening to give chase if we didn't.

To escape the enemy, we ran to the elevator and took it to the basement. As soon as the door opened and we tumbled out, we went running through the musty darkness alongside the dim chicken-wire storage rooms and the ever-glowing open mouth of the malevolent monster of a furnace. Bursting out the cellar door, we exited into the alley, once again safe to march and fight another day.

Exhausted but exhilarated, I would retreat to our apartment, where I would let Irwin wear my military equipment, while I tutored him in marching and singing military songs. This attention I paid to my brother pleased my mother, but she still drew the line at our marching on her newly waxed kitchen floor.

My longing for a uniform—and for some kind of outlet for my youthful energies—caught my father's attention. As the Allies took Paris in August, my father came home holding a large, long box under his arm. Placing it with great authority in my hands, he commanded me to open it. Inside the box was a brand-new, sharply creased Boy Scout uniform, complete with regulation belt, knee-high socks, pleated scarf, and lanyard.

"This is a uniform for you. And your black Thom McAn shoes," he signed, "with a good shine on them, will be perfect."

I did not know a single kid in all of Brooklyn who was a Boy Scout. *There must be a reason no one is in the Scouts,* I thought as I held the box in my arms.

While I stood there, my father marched (there is no other word for it) into his bedroom and returned, still marching, with a silver-framed picture of himself, taken when he was a boy. The picture showed him dressed in his deaf-school military uniform, peaked cap and all. The photo was dated 1912. He looked exactly like one of the Union drummer boys in the Civil War pictures that were in our history books at school.

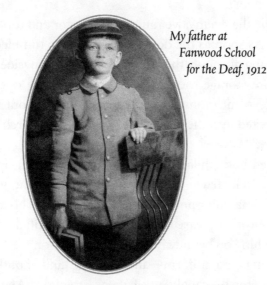

*My father at
Fanwood School
for the Deaf, 1912*

"You're just the same as I was when I was your age," he signed to me, emphasizing the sign for *same.* "I was easily bored, just like you. Left to myself, I would get into trouble of one kind or another. After all, I had no one to talk to. No one in my family knew sign. The kids on my block did not know sign. I was on my own.

However, that all changed when I went to Fanwood, my deaf residential school. It was patterned after a military academy and was run like a miniature version of West Point. We wore uniforms and marched constantly: from class to class, from class to dining hall, from dining hall to gymnasium, from gymnasium to playing fields, and virtually from pisspot to pisspot."

I had to ask him to explain his sign for *pisspot*. His two hands pointed downward, one in front of the other, pivoting at the wrists. I understood immediately. Then they moved back and forth—*marching*—his dangling fingers indicating the rows upon rows of marchers, stepping out in unison and in perfect harmony. Watching his hands, I was hypnotized; I could see my father and his schoolmates, rank upon rank, marching, marching, marching.

"You can't imagine what a good marcher I became, although at the time I saw no practical use in the Bronx for this odd skill. Unless you count marching in my dreams as a skill." He smiled at the thought.

And then like a cloudburst, my father's face suddenly darkened. "Later, I came to understand why the school placed so much emphasis on us deaf kids being disciplined. Our hearing teachers thought that being deaf, we would be uncontrollable if left to ourselves, like animals in the wild. So, their thinking went, we had to be disciplined—we had to be taught, basically, to obey orders. But that's another story."

Taking me by the hand, we *marched* into my bedroom, where my father watched as I put on my spanking-new, sharply creased Boy Scout uniform. *Now what?* I wondered.

As if reading my mind, my father signed, "The Boy Scouts are not big on marching. But discipline and obedience are important. And you could use a healthy dose of both. But don't worry, it's not all about that. You'll learn things as well. And for every new subject you master, you'll get a merit badge. I'll help you with that."

The first meeting was to be held in the basement of our scout leader's home, on the other side of Seth Low Park. Although it was just four blocks away, it might as well have been on the other side of the Atlantic Ocean. I was not in the habit of wandering far from my block.

For my first meeting my father accompanied me, waiting outside until it ended after a couple of hours. I had never been so bored in my life. All we did at that first den meeting was repeat, over and over again, the Boy Scout oath.

Subsequent meetings seemed to be no improvement. If anything they were worse because my father ceased to accompany me, which meant that every time I ventured out in my ridiculously elaborate blue uniform, the bullies in the neighborhood chased after me, making fun of me. But my father remained enthusiastic. He'd consulted the "merit badge" section of the Boy Scout manual and was determined that I should earn one.

So one night after supper I found myself at the kitchen table, sorting through about a million assorted postage stamps, spilled from a plastic bag that my father had bought in a philatelic shop in the city. Staring up at me were assorted strange-looking faces, covered in various styles of facial hair—spade whiskers, waxy curled mustaches, even muttonchops—and an equally exotic assortment of strange beasts, all printed in brilliant colors.

In the exact middle of the table sat a new stamp book, open to the first, blank page, which seemed to dare me to fill it, so as to one day earn my very first merit badge: "Stamp Collecting. MB [merit badge] No. 108."

My father put on his printer's visor, shielding his eyes from the kitchen light, and delicately selected a single stamp from the jumbled pile. Holding it carefully by the edge, he placed it in front of me, handed me a shovel-headed pair of tweezers and a hinge, and instructed me to mount the stamp in the appropriate-size box on the blank page of the stamp album.

I grasped the stamp with the sharp tweezers and pressed it onto the glued hinge—and in so doing, tore the whiskered face in half.

My father groaned. "Gently, softly." My father's hands gently, softly, and ever so slowly squeezed an invisible object.

I tried again. This effort produced an interesting crease in the otherwise curled horns of an antelope, creating the illusion that they grew out of the poor animal's tail.

In desperation, not waiting for my father's comment, I grabbed yet another of the pristine colored bits of paper and gently, softly, placed it squarely on the hinge in the dead center of a box. I paused, letting the glue dry and so adhere to page and stamp.

Satisfied that I had at last brought the process to a successful conclusion, I gently, softly, removed the tweezers—taking the entire perimeter of the stamp, now glued to the tweezers, along with it, and leaving the heart of the stamp defiantly glued to the hinge on the page.

Looking up, I saw my father's eyes cross, and his lips compress in anguish. His expressive hands lay silenced on top of his head. He had nothing to say.

I dug into that pile of stamps frantically, desperately, time and time again, with pretty much the same results.

Finally my father stilled my hands in his. "I have another idea," he signed.

The following week he brought home a set of X-Acto knife carving tools. Three knives were housed in individual black cushioned recesses in the bottom of a blond wood case. An assortment of extremely sharp-looking blades, of various sizes and shapes, were held in place by felt loops on the inside of the brass-hinged lid. The lid had an ornate brass latch that fit precisely into a matching brass catch. The whole affair was a wonder to my eyes. It was magnificent. But what in the world was it for? I wondered.

"MB No. 118. Wood Carving," my father signed to me, with an optimism I was sure was misguided.

That evening we sat, my father, brother, and I, where we always sat when there was a project at hand—at the kitchen table. And as usual my mother was doing the dinner dishes, her back turned to us, but a definite smile on her face; a smile that threatened, I thought, to break into a belly laugh.

The X-Acto knife set sat squarely in the middle of the table, on a sheet of the day's newspaper. Alongside the open case were three bars of Ivory soap.

"We'll break in these knives by carving the bars of soap. That way we won't dull the blades, and you'll get practice in carving."

That made sense to me, and picking up one of the knives, I proceeded to slice a bar of soap neatly in two, along with the web of skin between my thumb and forefinger.

My brother, who had been eyeing the box of blades enviously, left the table in a precipitous rush at the sight of the blood spurting from my hand. He was always complaining to my father that I always got new things first, never shared them, and passed them on to him only when they got old and worn or even broken. But this time he lost interest in my latest acquisition almost immediately.

Once the flow of blood was stemmed and the cut was bandaged, we tried again.

"Gently, softly," my father signed. I was frankly getting tired of these signs.

But slowly, gently, softly, I learned to use the knives and succeeded in carving out of the soft, yielding soap an approximation of an antelope. Sure, it looked as if its horns were growing out of its tail—actually, it looked remarkably like the stamp I had mangled. But what the heck, it wasn't half bad. *I can do this,* I thought.

"Practice," my father signed. I did. Every afternoon I carved an animal from a bar of soap, some strictly from my imagination, and every evening I would display the result to my mother and father, as my brother stared skeptically at my latest effort.

"WONDERFUL," my mother would sign expansively, exploding her open hands from the sides of her face in admiration.

"Practice," my father's more subdued sign suggested. I did. In time the bathroom was filled to overflowing with grotesque soap animals of every imaginable description. We washed with elephants with one ear missing. My brother and I bathed with mice and rats missing tails and ears. My father shaved with short-necked giraffes. And my mother did the dishes with soap nightmares that no one, not even myself, could explain. However, the scabs that formed on both of my hands, the result of countless nicks and cuts, were easily identifiable.

After about a hundred bars of Ivory soap—and a pint of blood, spilled drop by drop—we abandoned the project known as "MB No. 118. Wood Carving." And about a week after that my Boy Scout uniform was gently wrapped in tissue paper, mothballs, and cedar shavings and put away in the bottom drawer of my dresser. What was the use of being a Boy Scout, my father and I agreed, if I couldn't get even one darn merit badge?

My brother was thrilled. Here was something of mine, he realized, that would one day be passed down to him in virtually pristine condition. But by the time that day finally arrived, he had lost all interest. No one on our block was a Boy Scout, and for that matter, no one had *ever* been a Boy Scout. And my brother had no more interest than I did in being known as the first Boy Scout on West Ninth Street.

Memorabilia

A Chip Off the Old Block

Although my father's quest for a Boy Scout merit badge for me ultimately met with no more success than did the Brooklyn Dodgers' annual quest for the World Series, he was nonetheless determined that I follow in his footsteps and develop a passion for a hobby—any hobby.

My father had many hobbies, which was typical for the deaf of that time and place, as they had nothing like the breadth of entertainment available for the deaf today (most notably, captioned television and captioned DVDs). And my father became an expert in every hobby he ever tried.

My father was also a great believer in heredity. Thus, he reasoned, not only would I enjoy having a hobby, but like him I would excel at it. And so began a steady accumulation of "sets" brought home by my eager father, on which I was to hone my hobby skills.

My A.C. Gilbert Chemistry Set was housed in a cunning wooden case, secured by a brass catch. Inside the hinged double case were shelves containing an impressive array of chemicals in glass jars, many with cork stoppers, and trays of glass test tubes and tiny measuring spoons, litmus paper, and a spatula. There was even a small but effective balance and an alcohol lamp.

Each jar of chemicals had a label affixed to its side, with an exotic, often indecipherable name: phenolphthalein; ammonium chloride; sodium carbonate; sodium ferrocyanide;

cobalt chloride (a beautiful color); calcium oxide; ferric ammonium sulfate. On and on marched the jaw-dropping names across the rows of jars, neatly stacked in their wooden racks.

Accompanying this impressive collection of chemicals was a manual titled *Fun with Chemistry*. The cover displayed a young boy holding a lightning bolt.

My father instructed me to read the manual before I attempted any experiment. Then he left me to enjoy my new hobby, signing, "Have fun. Experiment."

I was a fast reader and soon scanned the two hundred–odd experiments that the manual promised were possible with the judicious use of the chemicals contained in this set.

The very next afternoon, with my mother's grudging permission, I set up my "lab" in our bathroom.

Closing the bathroom door behind me, imagining myself the mad scientist I had seen in last week's movie, I proceeded to do "experiments."

I turned water into "wine"—actually, clear water into rose-colored water.

I made writing ink, which was invisible until heated over my alcohol flame.

I exhausted the supply of litmus paper, transforming the various strips into a variety of stunning colors after dipping them in assorted toxic brews.

I was even able to create smoke, after mixing four different chemicals in a test tube, which rose to our bathroom ceiling and hung there like fog until I dispersed it with bathroom towels.

Then I got bored—until I recalled the boy holding the lightning bolt.

Impatiently putting aside the manual, I wondered what

would happen if I mixed certain chemicals, based just on their color and the sound of their names.

Mixing no fewer than twelve chemicals together, I applied the resulting mixture to the heat of my alcohol lamp. Standing in the tub, I watched from behind the shower curtain as the flame licked at the bottom of the test tube, held in its metal rack. Slowly but surely the mixture began to bubble—then boil. Then it exploded!

The paint peeled from the ceiling of our bathroom. The sound of exploding glass was deafening. But I had no problem in that respect, as I knew my mother had heard not a thing.

The smell was something else again. The stink was all-enveloping, the sulfurous odor of Hades itself.

One whiff of that scalding odor as it wafted from beneath the bathroom door, and my mother was at the door, yanking it open. Whereupon a huge cloud of smoke drifted into the living room, covering every piece of furniture, seeping into the fabric covering the couch, and eventually dying in the folds of the drapes hanging in front of our windows.

"*What in God's name,*" my father signed as he came through our front door that evening, "*is that horrible smell?*"

My mother quietly informed her husband that "his son" had been "experimenting." She couldn't help adding, "Just as you told him to."

A week after disposing of my A.C. Gilbert Chemistry Set, my father brought home an A.C. Gilbert Erector Set.

Opening it, I examined the multitude of metal girders in varying lengths, and assorted colored perforated metal pieces in all shapes and sizes, along with a multitude of nuts and bolts and washers. And there, held in a special slot, was an electric motor.

Accompanying all of it was, as usual, a detailed instruction manual. On the cover of the manual was a picture of a boy standing next to a huge Ferris wheel that stood well over his head, with swinging multicolored cars, the whole thing powered by an electric motor.

Holding that image firmly in mind—but not deigning to refer to any instructions contained inside the manual—I furiously began to assemble the girders and metal plates.

"God help me," my mother signed to me, as she watched me attaching girder to girder, every which way, never once looking at any instructions. "You remind me of my father, Max."

Now that was a surprise. I knew my mother's feelings for her father were, to say the least, complicated. And by now Celia, his long-suffering wife, had shown him the door for the last time. Having been taken in by Anne, the wife of my mother's youngest brother, Milton, he lived in Stony Creek, Connecticut—as different a place from Coney Island as the forests of Hungary were from the tenements of Manhattan Island. What on earth my mother saw in me that could even remotely make her think of him was beyond my grasp.

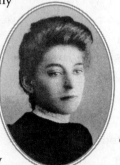

My mother's mother, Celia, circa 1902

Apparently, however, my last escapade had opened the floodgates of memory for my mother, prompting another story about her foolish father, Max the Gypsy, and his ever-practical wife, Celia, the thin-nosed, tight-lipped Russian beauty who hated him with undiluted passion.

"My father, Max, had only one job in his entire life," she signed to me. "And that job lasted but one day and ended with my father going to jail for a week." The sign for *jail* is quite explicit and would be understood by anyone: the two hands overlap in front of the face, fingers extended to form small openings; the eyes peek through the "bars." My impressionable young mind easily pictured my grandfather, Max, staring indignantly through the iron bars of his cell, while Celia stared back at him with the condemnatory look she reserved just for him. "Someone he knew got him a job as a pig-iron worker; pig iron was used in those days in the manufacturing of fire escapes, an item in great demand, as apartment buildings were sprouting up all over Brooklyn. Of course, Max knew nothing about the making of pig iron, but not knowing something was not the end of the matter for my father, only the beginning. And by beginning, I don't mean of the learning process but the bullshitting process."

My mother got her propensity for using the occasional scatological sign from my father, who not only loved them but in our home was the proud inventor of many.

"Max had no patience for instruction of any kind," my mother signed. "He preferred his native, forest-bred Gypsy intuitiveness. So with only a bare minimum of information, he began, with great energy and imagination, to mix his first batch of pig iron.

"Unfortunately, at that moment the owner of this modest Brooklyn version of a Pittsburgh steel mill strolled through the door, observed this ragged stranger mixing a brew unlike any he had ever seen, and promptly asked what the hell he thought he was doing.

"'Making pig iron, and who the hell are you?' my father answered.

"The owner called over the foreman and demanded an explanation.

"The foreman, not knowing much about my father and his Hungarian temper, denied any responsibility; whereupon my father picked up a lead pipe and smashed it over his head. Max would never tolerate injustice of any kind. As the unconscious foreman lay at his feet, and the owner stood staring at my father slack-jawed, Max said, with great dignity—as he later told Celia—'I quit!' And he added, 'Do your worst.' One week in the clink was what the state demanded as repayment from my father. A week he seemed proud to pay, in the cause of justice.

"My father never worked for anyone ever again. Instead he began a long career as a self-designated professional expert craftsman. His imagination far outstripped any skills he may have had, which in any case he lacked the patience to stop and acquire." My mother paused. "You remind me of him in that way.

"By turns my father was a roofer, then a plumber," she continued. "As a roofer, he walked backward off a roof while measuring it. As a plumber, he turned a gas valve *on*, rather than *off*, and almost gassed the entire neighborhood."

By now it was quite late in the afternoon. My father would be coming home from work within the hour. It was time for my mother to begin preparing the evening meal. My mother's hands stopped abruptly in midsentence and hung suspended in the gray light, thinking.

"Yes, in a way, you're a chip off the old block."

16
Brooklyn Bully

$\mathcal{F}$reddy was the bully of our block and the bane of my existence. He was the angriest kid in our neighborhood, maybe the angriest kid in all of Brooklyn. He was mad from sunup to sundown. Every kid in the neighborhood was his natural enemy. We sometimes wondered about this. What the heck was Freddy so angry about? What did we ever do to him?

If not for my speed, Freddy would have caught me during our weekly early-evening footraces across the grass and down the pathways of Seth Low Park, in the brief period when my father was still making me go to Boy Scout meetings. With the hated yellow scarf flying over my shoulder as he gained on me, I wished I were four inches taller and thirty pounds heavier. But I wasn't, and with that knowledge I increased my speed a notch, leaving him, gasping, behind. Safe again!

Freddy's goal, thus far unrealized, was to come upon me unawares and administer his infamous "Indian burn." Whenever Freddy caught a kid, always one smaller than himself, he would grab the boy's arm in his ham-hock hands, at its most tender part, and then twist, so that each fat hand went in the opposite direction from the other. The result was always the same: a mighty howl of pain from the unfortunate boy and a forearm as red as if it had been exposed to a Bunsen burner.

If the Indian burn failed to motivate the boy to sue for peace, Freddy administered his knuckle rap: a short, sharp *pang* on the head with his pointed knuckle, which was, unlike his hand, fat free and thus quite pointy. For the unfortunate boy who had a crewcut, this procedure raised an interestingly shaped knot on his head, often the size of an egg. Such was the outcome of Freddy catching you.

As I was the only kid on our block who had so far escaped Freddy's ministrations, I held a special place in his malignant heart. He could not catch me, as I easily outran him. And when trapped, as in an alley, I was agile enough that I could squirm my way to safety. This drove him crazy. Especially when, just out of his reach, I would laugh and taunt him. This proved to be my undoing.

Freddy was not a stupid boy. He was a bit fat and clumsy perhaps, and slow-footed for sure, but he was not slow-witted. I could outrun him, but there was always the possibility that he could outthink me. Freddy developed a plan—a plan to silence my jeering insults and end my humiliating escapes, perhaps forever.

The tar-paper roof of our apartment house, accessed through a heavy metal door, was my private park, as I've said, the one place on our busy Brooklyn block where I could go and be completely by myself. I had obtained a copy of the primitive key that secured the door. It was my most precious possession. With it I could remove myself from the incessant noise and activity that permeated my block. I could sit, my back to the low perimeter of the brick roof wall, and read a book, or wonder about my life, or just look at the clouds sailing by in the blue sky over Brooklyn. And from my roof, on a really clear day, I could catch glimpses of the Atlantic

Ocean reflecting the early-morning light, lying off Coney Island, just a few miles away.

Needless to say, I sometimes let my guard down during these reveries, and one fateful afternoon that almost led to my undoing.

Unbeknownst to me, Freddy had studied my movements over the course of a typical week, the better to plan my eventual capture. Having made careful note of my sudden and inexplicable disappearances, he followed silently behind as I took myself to the roof one day.

Usually I used my secret key to relock the metal roof door behind me as soon as I got there. But on this particular afternoon, in my haste to read a new book, I forgot.

Deeply engrossed in the predicament of the main character, I failed to hear Freddy creeping up on me. When I finally heard his sneakered feet sliding over the graveled roof, it was almost too late.

Leaping to my feet, I threw my book at his head and ran past him, as he reflexively ducked. It was a thick book. It contained many chapters, many adventures. Had I been reading a thin, insubstantial comic book, my fate would have been sealed.

But my reprieve was brief. I dashed to the roof door, only to discover that Freddy had jammed it shut. I then ran, like a demented rat in a maze, all around the roof. Through and around the sheets hanging from the clotheslines on the roof, around the twin chimney stacks, and around the many protruding air vents that jutted up from the roof, I raced, with Freddy in close pursuit.

Slowly but surely Freddy herded me into a corner. I was trapped.

The next thing I knew, I was dangling, head down, held only by my ankles, over the edge of the roof.

Strangely, I was not afraid. Instead I was fascinated, in an odd way, to observe the ground six floors below my head. I had, literally, a bird's-eye view of the clotheslines extending from each apartment window. Now, I thought, if Freddy were to let me go, I would bounce off the clotheslines, as a steel ball bounces off the many bumpers on a pinball machine before ending its journey—in the slot at the bottom of the machine—without a scratch.

I couldn't help wondering where I would end up if dropped. But since I was not a steel ball and was unlikely to end without a scratch, I dismissed *that* question from my mind.

As I had a wonderful imagination, a new image, unbidden, came clearly to mind: on the way down I would be trapped in one of the giant brassieres hanging from Mrs. Abromovitz's line.

It's remarkable how your imminent demise so sharply focuses your mind. I could visualize in acute detail the shocked look on Mrs. Abromovitz's face as she unsuspectingly reeled me in along with the rest of her wash. The image so amused me that I burst into laughter.

This laugh was to be my salvation. Hearing me, Freddy thought that he had failed to scare the wits out of me. Never having actually intended to drop me (I hoped), he pulled me back onto the roof.

Thereafter Freddy never bothered me again. He had done his worst, and I had laughed in his face. He had never before encountered such bravery. I had passed some insane test that only he could devise. I was the envy of every kid on the block.

17
Polio

Nineteen forty-five was the height of the polio scare in America. And so it was that every mother in Brooklyn forced down her children's throats a daily dose of cod-liver oil. The sickening, vile, thick, oily, fishy-smelling liquid clung to our lips, coated our tongues, and lined our throats for hours. It was impossible to get rid of the taste. We resigned ourselves to the fact that it just had to wear off by itself, in its own sweet time.

"It's good for you," my mother signed, in exasperation at our daily struggle; often, she literally had to force my mouth open for my daily dose. I hated most fish, and I despised cod-liver oil, the deadliest by-product of fish ever devised by man—pure distilled evil, as far as I was concerned.

My brother, on the other hand, was used to taking medicine every day to control his seizures and not only took it without complaint but may even have liked it.

"It hurts me more than it does you," my mother signed after our daily dose had been administered.

Then came the killer ending to any argument: "Do you want to get polio?"

We Brooklyn boys and girls heard about polio what seemed like every day of our lives, especially in the summertime. For us kids, summer was the golden time, wonderful carefree days blending seamlessly one into the other. But for our parents it was another matter entirely: "Don't get overheated. Do you want to get polio?" (This was invariably followed by "That's what happened to President Roosevelt when he was a young man. Do you want to sit in a wheelchair for the rest of your life like him?") "Don't go in the water right after eating. You'll get a cramp and die. And if not, you'll get polio." "Stay away from crowds. You'll get polio." "Don't get dirty. You'll get polio." "You can't go to the movies this Saturday. Some kid on the next block got polio." "Don't drink at the public fountain. You'll get polio." "Don't eat food if a fly lands on it. You'll get polio." *Don't do this, don't do that.* And then the dreaded final words: "Do you want to end up in an iron lung?"

Because she wanted to emphasize that this was a matter that went beyond her daily and wide-ranging litany of prohibitions, my mother employed not the usual one but two signs for *don't.* She used the everyday, utilitarian *don't* that she employed for any number of ordinary occasions, whenever I was doing something she preferred me not to be doing—the quick flick of her thumb from under her chin. And then, to leave no room for doubt or argument, she used the special *don't* with crossed hands, palms facing me, which she would repeatedly separate and recross, all the while looking at me with the sternest expression she could muster.

She would keep it up until I acknowledged her warnings to her satisfaction—not with a simple nod of my head or a shake of my hinged fist in the sign for *yes,* but with an emphatically finger-spelled "Okay! Okay! . . . OKAY, ALREADY!"

And if I ever, heaven forbid, had a sniffle, or a stomachache, she put me to bed immediately; and until the sniffle or the stomachache was gone, and I had convinced her that it was, she hovered over me, like a soft enveloping cloud.

My brother was even more closely monitored. Whenever there was a reported outbreak of polio, she would keep him indoors, always at her side, so that there wasn't even the slightest chance of his being exposed to polio—or any other germ, for that matter.

No one knew how a person got polio; our doctor didn't, the scientists didn't, our teachers didn't, and our parents didn't. Even Mrs. Birnbaum, who spied on the entire block while leaning out of her bedroom window all day long with her fat arms resting on a pillow, didn't, and she knew *everything*. But our parents seemed convinced that heat was a great incubator of the polio germ, and they viewed the long golden days of summer with particular alarm. Every time a heat wave descended on Brooklyn, all the kids in the neighborhood were consigned to their rooms.

As I was performing my magic tricks for my brother in our bedroom one day, I wondered: If an epileptic person caught polio, would his seizures stop? Like magic? I also wondered: Were deaf people perhaps immune to the disease? I had never heard of a deaf person who had polio. My father hadn't either. "We have enough trouble without polio," he signed when I asked him about it. "Maybe God has spared us."

But God did not spare Barry Goldstein, my friend from across the street. Late that summer, just as we were feeling the first hints of fall in the air and thinking that the danger might be over for the season, a blast of heat drove the cool air off. At the height of this last heat wave, Barry got sick. And his sickness became polio. Now I knew someone who had polio.

Barry was taken to Coney Island Hospital and was immediately put into an iron lung. For the next few weeks it was touch and go, but finally he stabilized. The iron lung did his breathing for him.

One day Barry's father came to our apartment door with a

handwritten note for my father: "You and Myron can visit my son if you want. I think he'd like that."

The very next Saturday my father and I took the subway to Coney Island, and then we walked to the hospital. My father did not sign a single sign to me. There was nothing he could say to me that would lessen my shock at my friend's illness and the sadness of his condition.

Coney Island Hospital seemed the stuff of nightmares to us kids. We'd heard about people going there, but they never seemed to come out. We were sure it was the place where you went to die. Once my father and I arrived, its appearance more than lived up to my worst fears: dark, dank hallways, cheerless gray rooms filled wall to wall with beds inhabited by ghastly looking sick people.

The elevator took us to the top floor, where we exited onto a dark hallway. At the far end was a single large room, blindingly illuminated by numerous hanging lights. In the room were row upon row of iron lungs, lined up in neat columns. Protruding from the end of each one was a solitary head resting on a pillow. Above each head was a tilted mirror. By looking at this mirror, each patient could see what lay immediately behind him.

Looking in his mirror, Barry saw me. And looking in the same mirror, I saw Barry's upside-down face—and watched him smile at me.

Only Barry's head was visible. The rest of him lay hidden in the iron lung.

Barry and I had a good visit. I told him about all the happenings on the block since he had gotten sick. (I didn't once mention the word *polio*.) Some of my stories made him laugh.

He told me I could ride his bike until he came home and could use it himself.

Soon a nurse came by and ushered us out, telling us, "This boy needs his rest."

We said our goodbyes, and as I was leaving, he said, "You know, I have polio."

On the way home in the subway car, my father signed to me his sadness. "Poor, poor boy."

But then he signed something surprising. "Now I know why I never heard of a deaf person getting polio." He paused, thinking. "God wouldn't do that to a deaf person. How would a deaf person talk, if his hands were hidden in an iron lung? How would a deaf person sign his fears with hidden hands?" My father did not sign an additional thought all the way home.

That fall it rained almost every day. Barry's bike sat on his porch, exactly where he had left it after his last ride, a mute reminder of my friend. It was never taken in when it rained, and by the beginning of winter it was covered in rust. With winter's first snowfall, it disappeared completely under a layer of snow, which meant that now when I looked over at his silent white porch as I left my apartment building each morning, the image of Barry in his iron lung, unable to ride his bike, no longer leaped unbidden into my mind.

For my father, however, the thought of polio was much on his mind all that winter, as was his God, the god who would inflict polio on a young boy.

I had no interest in God as represented by the dilapidated wooden synagogue around the corner from us, with its smelly, impossibly foreign-looking men dressed in the same drab black clothing year round. This mysterious exclusive gathering was the world of my father's father, not mine. My world was the *moment*, as represented by my Brooklyn block, not a history five thousand years old.

But I was never clear how my father felt about this subject. Our family did not observe the Sabbath. We did not keep any

Jewish holidays, as many—though not all—of my Jewish friends did. Although my father had had a bar mitzvah—an experience, he told me, that was totally incomprehensible to him—he knew no prayers. He did not attend weekly services at our neighborhood synagogue, or even High Holy Day services. What would have been the point? He could not sing the hymns, nor read the words. God did not speak to him, and if He did, my father could not hear Him. There were no signs known to the deaf for the ancient Hebrew words, so how could he speak to God, in God's language?

My father talked to me about everything, but not his God. One day, however, my father came home early from work. There was a

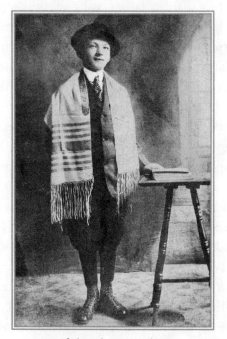

My father's bar mitzvah, 1915

snowstorm, and he had been given a half-day off with pay, as the paper supply had been exhausted, and fresh newsprint inventory was stuck on trucks stranded in snowdrifts north of the city. As usual, he had the day's paper folded under his arm, but there was not much to it since there was no sports news (thanks to the snowstorm), no reports of murders the night before in Brooklyn (probably for the same reason), and very little in the way of war news (fortunately). Lacking any news to discuss with me, and being in an unaccountably thoughtful mood, my father began, that afternoon, a halting monologue about the role God had played in his life.

"My father was a deeply religious man from the old country," he signed to me. "And in the old country his father was a cantor. I was told as a boy that my father had a sweet voice. I have some memory of this, but I can never pin it down in my mind. I remember him covering himself every morning with his shawl, and then wrapping his arm and forehead with his tefillin, which he kept in a burgundy velvet bag embroidered in heavy gold thread with Hebrew words." My father's sign for *Hebrew* was clear: his two hands descended downward from his chin repeatedly, opening and closing as if stroking a long imaginary beard. "Then my father would bend up and down repeatedly, and talk to someone; someone I couldn't see, but who was in the room with us. I knew he was talking, because I saw his lips moving, moving, moving.

"But as observant a Jew as my father was, when I was a boy he never involved me in his daily rituals. And how could he? We never talked. We had no real language.

"So I never knew who God was. It was a mystery all my life. Still is. Like everything else for us deaf, life is a puzzle, and we have only ourselves to solve the thousands of pieces of the puzzle." While he was telling me this, his fingers revolved around each other, as if they were manipulating pieces of a jigsaw puzzle, a giant ever-changing puzzle that only he could see. Then my father looked at me for the longest time. "Sometimes I *hate* God. He made me deaf, but not my sisters or my brother. Why was that? I was only a little boy. What did I do wrong? I never understood. And now look at your friend Barry. Such a sweet boy. He always smiles at me and tries to sign *hello* to me. Now he will never ride his bike again. Why would God do such a thing?

"And what kind of god would cause your brother, a sweet beautiful boy who never hurt anyone, to be an epileptic? Why did God strike him so? Does God see him when he falls down? Does God care when he bites his tongue and his blood flies everywhere?"

My father expected no answer from me. He sat there at the kitchen table, deeply troubled. I could read it on his face and in the slump of his shoulders. For the longest time my father continued to stare into space, lost in the maze of unanswerable questions, until I saw him slowly begin to refocus. He was looking at me with a strange expression on his face, and his hands began to move.

"But just when I curse God, I think of Mother Sarah. I think of you and your brother. And I think this puzzle will never be answered."

Memorabilia

The End of the Presidency

On April 12, 1945, President Franklin Delano Roosevelt died unexpectedly in Warm Springs, Georgia. He had looked increasingly old, weary, and sad as the war dragged on. But as he was the only president I had ever known, his death was shocking news to me. That night, as always, my father brought home the newspaper. After supper he signed the front-page headline: "FDR DEAD." His sign was as bold and black as was the bold, black-printed headline. My father's hands were sad and mournful. "He was a cripple. He had polio as a young man. Until then he was just like any other young man." Then he stopped. "I was just like any other boy, until I got sick. Then I was crippled in my ears, just like the president was crippled in his legs. But look what FDR could do. He won the war."

Then my father cried. I had never seen my father cry before. He did not make a newspaper hat from the front page that night.

18
A Boy Becomes a Man

On August 6, 1945, a lone American plane dropped a single bomb on the city of Hiroshima, signaling the end of World War II.

One month earlier, the day after I turned twelve, my father had dropped a bomb on me. He informed me that I would have my bar mitzvah when I was thirteen, a year later. That news was as shocking to me as the news of the atomic bomb. Bar mitzvah? Since when, I wondered, was my father interested in the traditions of the Jewish religion? Until the day he spoke to me about his sense of alienation from God, I'd never gotten the impression that religion occupied any space, positive or negative, in his thoughts.

Although born of Jewish parents, he had had no formal Jewish upbringing, unless you counted the mock bar mitzvah he had undergone. All he remembered of that event, he told me, was being unaccountably dressed in a suit and hat one Saturday upon turning thirteen, and accompanying his father to the local *shul*, the storefront house of worship. There he was pushed onto a wooden stage, where he stood with a prayer shawl draped around his shoulders and a man's hat on his head. Then he watched carefully, but with a total lack of comprehension, while the gray-bearded rabbi faced him, his hair-shrouded lips moving, my father said, a mile a minute.

"I had no idea," he told me, "what was going on. No one could explain it to me, and no one even bothered to try. Like much of my life in the hearing world at that age, nothing I experienced made much sense."

My grandfather had reasoned that as his firstborn son could not hear, he could never truly participate in any formal religious services. Of the Torah, did not Moses instruct the priests to "read it in their ears"? Being deaf, how could his son hear Torah? And as God did not speak in sign, how would God hear him respond? And so it was that my father had his bar mitzvah in silence; it was a dumb show, devoid of all meaning. My father's final word on the subject was the observation that during the ceremony, he saw tears falling from his father's eyes, disappearing into his beard. Tears of joy? Tears of sadness? My father could not say.

But now, to the surprise of both sides of the family, my father was determined that his firstborn son, their firstborn grandchild, would have a bar mitzvah. He would show them all that even though he was a deaf father, he knew how to raise a hearing son in the proper fashion and that, in all the ways that counted, he was as good a father as any hearing father.

All the long year that followed, surely the longest year of my young life, I endured my weekly bar mitzvah lessons. It was a dreary year of rote, uncomprehending chanting done to the metronomic tune of the rabbi's rod-cane beating on my desktop, with occasional well-directed swipes at my knuckles as I stumbled over a particularly grievous passage. Slogging my undistinguished way through my lessons, I found the experience sheer torture.

But when I finally stood at the podium of our local synagogue reading my Torah section, and then recited my "Today I Am a Man" speech, my father's face beamed up at me from the front row of the congregation with a look of undisguised pride—a pride not in the least diminished by the fact that he had not heard a single word I spoke. That made it all worthwhile. Although his hands never once moved from his lap to explain how he felt, his face said it all. Just as his father had done so many years in the past, my father was quietly crying.

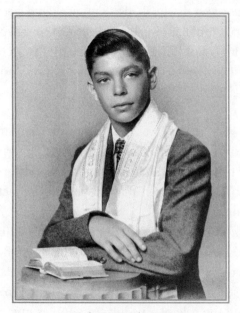

My bar mitzvah, 1946

As for me, the bar mitzvah boy, it seemed to me that the only result I experienced as a consequence of my year-long enforced brush with piety was an amazing increase in speed. I could run like the wind.

You see, as a "Jewish adult man" in the eyes of Jewish tradition, I was now eligible to complete the ten-man *minyan* necessary for the daily service at the synagogue, which often didn't attract the requisite number. Thus in the midst of playing a game on our block, my friends and I would suddenly be interrupted by eight spry congregants sent out by the rabbi to scour the neighborhood for a recent bar mitzvah boy to complete the *minyan:* I was their latest target. I could almost hear their excited whispers as the pious Jews, older in years but still fleet of foot, rounded the corner and locked eyes on me: the newly minted bar mitzvah boy. My head start of a bare few yards never diminished as my sneakered feet pounded up the block, a gaggle of flapping long black coats in hot pursuit. They were surprisingly fast, but they never caught me. In time they focused their raids on newer, and slower, bar mitzvah boys.

*N*ow that I was a "man," I was officially grown up. Although I had always been old as a child because of my role as interpreter for my father in the hearing world, I was now fiercely determined to be grown up, to be considered mature beyond my actual years. I thought I had earned it.

My father continued to see me as an adult only when he needed me to be one. Most of the time I was still his child. But whenever we encountered a hearing-deaf situation in the outside, hearing world, I was still obliged to metamorphose into an instrument for his use and fill the role of an adult. As soon as my father's needs had been met, I morphed back into a child once again.

It was a dizzying transformation—child-adult-instrument-child—a veritable high-wire act, from which I could never look down, for fear of falling. And nothing about it was made easier by the fact that I was now a *man*, the rabbi having said so.

*W*hen my brother turned thirteen, there would be no bar mitzvah for him. My father's tenuous hold on religion, and his sense of himself as a Jewish father, had been discharged with my bar mitzvah. That occasion ended all formal connection with his mysterious God (until the cold drizzly day forty-two years later when he would be buried in a Jewish cemetery in Brooklyn, next to the graves of his mother and father). As before we kept no Sabbath in our Brooklyn apartment and attended no High Holy Day services in the wooden synagogue around the corner. And after my bar mitzvah, I never attended a single Saturday morning service in all the years I lived in Brooklyn.

I knew of my father's tortured relationship with his God. As a boy, I saw my father and my mother and their deafness, and I had my own angry questions for Him. These questions only multiplied when I saw how my brother suffered from epilepsy. Eventually I stopped caring. This God did not care about my family, and I would not care about Him.

19

Vaudeville on 86th Street

*A*fter the war ended, once a month my mother would lead my father, brother, and me to my grandmother Celia's apartment on 86th Street in Brooklyn. There all of her children and grand-children would gather for a Sunday dinner, at which we gave thanks for the safe return of my mother's brothers, Milton and Harry. Milton had been a paratrooper, stranded in the steaming jungles of Burma, where he had come down with malaria; Harry had been a sailor on the *USS Missouri,* the site of the signing of the unconditional surrender of Japan, which he witnessed firsthand, on the deck of his own ship. We had won the war, just as my father said we would. And now they were both home.

When we arrived at Celia's, my mother would immediately go to the kitchen—from which the most amazing odors were ema-nating—to help her mother and younger sister, Mary, cook the feast that they had been preparing all the previous week. The chicken had been plucked and was in the oven, the brisket lay marinating in a roasting pan, and an enormous cow's tongue sat simmering in a pot on the stove; now all that was left were the finishing touches—each of which "touches" for anyone else would constitute an entire meal for a family of four.

My brother and I quickly joined our cousins who, having traveled the farthest, usually arrived first. My favorite cousin was Stephen, my uncle David's son, who was just a few months younger than I. Stephen was nothing like me—he was tall and slim, where I was of average height and more muscular. He was fair-skinned and blond, where I was dark-haired and swarthy in complexion; in the summer I tanned, while he sunburned. He swam, as did his father, like a fish, while I resembled, like my father, an anchor in the water. Where he was extroverted, I was introspective. In short, as opposites in every way, we were perfectly suited to be the best of friends and, we assumed, friends for life.

While the cousins played, my father would join my mother's brothers David, Harry, and Milton, where he would promptly produce a pipe from his jacket pocket and begin elaborate preparations for a fresh bowlful of Walnut tobacco. Although my father was deaf and his brothers-in-law knew not a single word of sign language, within minutes of greeting one another they were deep in discussion—of a sort. This "discussion" consisted of exaggerated speech on their part, and sheer guesswork involving lipreading on my father's part. The misunderstandings that this area of "discussion" produced were comical, even more so because my father, being a comedian at heart, often exaggerated his malapropisms.

Politics was a subject of particular interest to my father and Milton, my mother's youngest brother. Because of his experience growing up poor during the Great Depression, Milton held strong beliefs on the superiority of an egalitarian, socialist society over the dog-eat-dog ways of capitalism, and before the war he had fought in Spain as part of the anti-Francoist Abraham Lincoln

Brigade. The other two brothers weren't much interested in politics. David, the oldest, was known far and wide in Brooklyn as "the Duke of Coney Island," and as I later learned, his interests lay basically in wine, women, and song. Harry, the middle brother, was as taciturn as his famously taciturn mother and betrayed no apparent interest in any subject whatsoever, least of all politics.

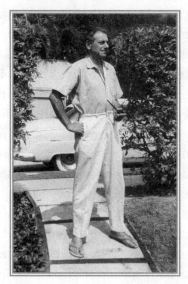

My mother's oldest brother, David, the Duke of Coney Island

But David and Harry were both fascinated by the lengthy political conversations between my father and Milton, not because of the content (which was slight) but because of the manner in which they conducted these pseudo-debates. Lacking a common language, my father and Milton communicated in mime. Of course, my father was the more gifted in this physical language, but Milton managed to hold his own—if not in technique, surely in inventiveness, enthusiasm, and conviction. One of the recurring bits involved pipe smoking.

All three of my mother's brothers were pipe smokers. No

sooner did my father put his empty pipe in his mouth than they followed suit. There they sat, thoughtful looks on their faces, four men with pipes in their mouths, staring expectantly straight ahead, like an ad for Walnut tobacco, the premier pipe tobacco of its day. However, in this case only my father had Walnut tobacco in his tobacco pouch. The others had rough-cut, no-name brands of lesser quality.

This frozen tableau was broken when my father began to load his pipe. The sweet aroma of his fine-cut tobacco caused his brothers-in-law's nostrils to flare, as they sniffed the air expectantly. When my father completed the task of lovingly tamping down the tobacco in his pipe bowl, Milton waved his empty pipe in front of my father's face. My father studiously ignored him.

Then my father ever so slowly lit his pipe with a wooden match and drew deeply. Holding that first mouthful of smoke within his bulging cheeks for the longest time, he opened his eyes wide, curled his lips up around the pipe stem in exaggerated satisfaction—and winked, all the while looking at Milton and shaking his head no.

I knew my father to be the most generous of men, so I understood that his broad gesture of refusal to accede to Milton's request was only the opening gambit—triggered by the political concept of "sharing"—of a prolonged discussion of the relative merits of Stalinist Russia and its Communist system, versus Harry Truman's self-reliant America, all done in mime, worthy of the opening act in a Coney Island vaudeville show.

Milton, taking his cue, acted out the sharing of his inferior tobacco with his two brothers, making it clear to my father that they got their bowlfuls before he got his. This was to symbolize the Soviet principle of sharing; one for all, and all for one. Then to underscore the point, only after his brothers had lit their pipes did Milton light his—with a *paper* match, the people's match.

Unfortunately, even after repeated attempts, his matches wouldn't light.

Taking the paper matches from Milton, my father, in broad gestures, struck match after match under Milton's nose, making sure that they would sputter but never light. Once he'd exhausted Milton's pack of proletarian paper matches, he dismissively made the sign for the hammer and sickle in Milton's face, scowling in perfect imitation of the photograph of Joseph Stalin at Yalta.

Begging a kitchen match from David, Milton lit his pipe. He drew on his pipe until his cheeks bulged, then blew a cloud of smoke in my father's direction. As the acrid odor of Milton's burning pipe tobacco passed in front of my father's nose, he gagged and grabbed his throat. As his eyes turned up in his head, he collapsed into the waiting arms of David and Harry.

Watching this pantomime, Stephen and I, along with our younger cousins, would run to my father with handkerchiefs, cushions, and pages from the Sunday newspaper, waving them in his face, attempting to revive him.

After a dramatic moment or two, my father would sit back up on the couch, draw a deep breath, smile, and in a show of East-West solidarity, offer his tobacco pouch to Milton.

The meal itself was the second act of this vaudeville show.

Since Celia had long ago exiled her philandering husband, Max, from her home, my father, being the oldest male in the family, was granted the right of *seigneur*, a role he played with broad comedic strokes. Sitting with great dignity at the head of the table, he would begin by pressing the edge of the carving knife against the ball of his thumb to test for sharpness, which of course brought forth gasps from my younger cousins. Then tilting his head sideways, he proceeded to perform a maneuver in which he appeared to insert the knife into his mouth (shielding most of the action with his opposite hand and a napkin), while his Adam's apple jerked up and down like a fishing bob with a hooked fish at the other end. Withdrawing his blade, he turned back to the table, and with his tongue flattened, he opened his mouth wide, revealing an empty dark cavern. I had seen my father perform this act many times, but he was so expert at it that even I could believe that he had cut off his tongue with the sharp carving knife—and then swallowed it. The sight of the large inert cow's tongue, severed at its root, lying lifeless on a platter in front of him, probably reinforced the illusion. Then my father winked and proceeded to carve the tip of the cow's tongue and place it in his mouth. While we sat mesmerized, he began to chew. After a moment of exaggerated chewing motions, he opened his mouth and ever so slowly stuck out his tongue, now magically restored.

The table broke into applause. Only Celia and Harry sat stone still, their faces as inexpressive as the granite ones carved into Mount Rushmore. Celia had the thinnest lips of any adult I ever knew, lips as straight and rigid as the edge of a ruler. As a child she had walked the muddy roads in the Pale of Russia, while being told that the streets of America were paved in gold. After hearing this fabulous story for years, one day she embarked, alone, for America. Immediately upon arriving in the Lower East Side of New York, her uneducated but acutely observant mind informed her that the streets of America were not paved in gold but rather were covered in horseshit. She did not have much to say for the rest of her life. And the only sweetness she allowed herself to experience was the lump of sugar she held between her teeth as she sipped her tea from an old jelly glass.

Moving into the next act, after the meal had been consumed—minus tongue for us kids who, after my father's performance, wanted no part of that vile organ—the men and children went to the living room, while my mother and her sister cleared the table. Once my father was settled, he would make four-cornered hats from the pages of the Sunday newspaper for us kids. Then, staring appraisingly at each of his brothers-in-law, he would affect an air of studious concentration, until he had his *aha* moment and began to make a hat for each of them.

The making of a newspaper hat involves some twenty-five well-executed steps. In the process of transmuting a flat, one-dimensional sheet of newsprint into a three-dimensional newspaper hat, various possibilities appear along the way.

At step fourteen, my father produced a pirate hat. Placing it with authority on his head, he formed his hands into a pistol and proceeded to empty Milton's pockets. Once Milton's pockets had been turned inside out, the pirate hat was placed on *his* head. Bereft of all possessions, Milton was now a pirate as well and could similarly *steal* the possessions of others. My father had made his political point.

Taking another sheet of newsprint, he again applied himself to the folding and scoring process. Step fifteen consisted of turning the pirate's hat sideways, so that it was now a bishop's miter. Solemnly making the sign of the cross, he took the hat over to Harry—who had married an Italian Catholic girl—and put it on his head. Then, placing a linen napkin on the floor, he knelt at Harry's feet, kissed Harry's wedding ring, and bowed his head, beseeching Harry's blessing. More from the desire to take the spotlight off himself than to engage in my father's nonsense, Harry made a lame version of the benediction.

My father picked up another page from the Sunday paper. This time he selected a page from the comics and began folding. At step sixteen, he held a perfectly formed sailor hat in his hand. Turning it this way and that, he admired the colorful hat, then placed it, at a rakish angle, on David's head. The Duke of Coney Island understood the gesture perfectly.

Harry, who failed to see any humor in all this, promptly removed his hat, but the other two brothers wore their hats for the rest of the afternoon. Milton would, from time to time, form his own hand pistol and demand money from my brother, whose pockets had been loaded with change by my father so that this scene could be performed all afternoon long—to my brother's great delight.

David loved his sailor hat and all that it implied, and he would pester his wife, Sylvia, for kisses and hugs, like any self-respecting sailor on shore leave in Coney Island. She, much annoyed and not thinking his importuning in the least amusing, would firmly push him away.

Since my mother's brothers had very little in common (except that all three had married outside the Jewish faith, as had my mother's sister), they gladly allowed my father to stay center stage at these family gatherings, directing his various vaudeville playlets. This relieved them of the obligation to find something to talk about. My father, in turn, figured that his antics took the pressure off my mother to attempt to create the illusion of familial unity—an impossible task for the deaf daughter of a hearing family, none of whom knew a single sign.

But my father had another reason for producing these performances. He once explained to me that it was a matter of control.

"When I'm with Mother Sarah's family," he told me, "I have no idea what's going on. Oh, they smile at me and talk to me, mouthing words as if I were an idiot, but we never have a real conversation. Then after a while they turn away from me and talk to each other, and I'm left feeling like a piece of furniture. But when I take charge, when I act out my little scenes with them, *I'm* in control, and I always know what's going on." Then he added, "And it's fun playing the clown sometimes. As long as it's on my terms."

One Sunday there was a new and unexpected act in the monthly comedic playlet, one that my father did not direct or star in. And rather than his usual fare of farce and comedy, this one was a bit of melodrama.

On that afternoon my cousin Stephen arrived late—without his mother—and without saying a word, he dropped a fat envelope in his father's lap. Turning quickly, he left my grandmother's apartment and closed the door solidly behind him. The envelope contained the divorce papers that David's wife was now serving on him.

I never saw Stephen, my friend for life, ever again.

20

Sounds from the Heart

*A*lthough he was deaf, my father could make vocal sounds; there was nothing wrong with his larynx. I can still vaguely remember the sounds he made when he was happy, and the sounds of grief that poured out of him at the news of President Roosevelt's death. But the single explosive sound of fear he made one evening, the only time I ever knew my father to be afraid, is seared in memory to this day.

It was early evening, and I was waiting for my father to finish his bath before my mother came home. She had gone to Coney Island to visit her mother and sister.

As I played with my newspaper hat and tried to make one for my brother, my father's deaf voice shattered the heavy stillness of our usually silent apartment, bringing me instantly to my feet. He screamed, again and again, the screams colliding with each other, bouncing off the tile walls of our small bathroom until they were one huge all-enveloping sound of pain.

I ran to my father, who was lying naked in the tub covered in blood. A shampoo bottle had shattered when he dropped it as he was getting out of the tub. In reaching down for it, he had slipped and fallen on a jagged shard of glass. Blood was pouring from a slab-size flap of skin that hung obscenely from his arm. Wherever I looked, I saw his bright red blood coating every white tile surface of the room.

With one hand my father held the slippery, hanging red flap in place, while his other hand signed for me to get the towel, his every movement flinging more blood from his gaping wound. I understood and wrapped the towel as tightly as I could around his arm while he held the flap in place. My father gathered the ends of the towel and twisted them into a loose knot, effectively creating a tourniquet that slowed his loss of blood. My brother stood at the bathroom door, looking on at the bloody scene in horror.

Furiously I stomped on the bathroom floor. Mrs. Abromovitz, our downstairs neighbor, recognized immediately that this was a signal of emergency and not the usual foot-stamping that our deaf family used to gain one another's attention. An ambulance soon arrived. I accompanied my father to serve as usual as his transla-tor, and I brought my brother with us, as I was afraid that if left alone in our empty apartment, he might have a seizure after all the excitement.

The emergency attendant who ministered to my father's wound on the way to Coney Island Hospital directed all his ques-tions to me as soon as he understood that my father was deaf.

"How did this happen?" he asked me in the back of the ambu-lance, as we careened around corners and sped down the streets of Brooklyn.

I asked my father.

"He slipped in the bathtub and fell on broken glass," I inter-preted.

"Ask your father how much blood he's lost."

I asked my father.

"How the hell should I know?" he answered me with one hand,

while holding on to the blood-drenched towel with the other. "Is this guy an idiot?"

"A lot," I told the attendant.

"Ask your father what his blood type is."

I asked my father.

"This guy *is* an idiot," my father responded with absolute disgust.

"My father wants to know, what are the choices?"

"A, B, or O," the attendant said.

I told my father his choices.

"Tell this fool to shove his choices up his ass," my father signed. "It's all alphabet soup to me. Just get me to a doctor!"

I could feel my own blood rising into my face and turning it bright red. I stiffened with shame.

"He's not sure," I said.

As soon as we pulled up to the ambulance entrance of the hospital, I was told to go to the admissions office, while my father was rushed into the emergency room.

For over an hour I tried to supply the answers to the multitude of questions asked of me about my father.

"Is your father deaf?"

"Yes."

"Can he hear if we speak loudly?"

"No, he is deaf."

"Can he hear if we shout?"

I didn't bother answering. This question had been asked of me many times when I was in public with my father. When I answered, "No, he is deaf," hearing people would often then shout at him over and over. When he didn't respond, they would walk off in disgust.

"Stupid hearing people," my father always said to me when this happened. "Pay no attention to them."

"Where does your father work? Does he have insurance? Do you have a telephone? Do you have a mother? Is she deaf? What's her name? How can we reach her?"

On and on it went. I answered as best I could.

"How come you can hear?"

I couldn't understand what that had to do with anything.

"How old are you?"

That one I answered with no problem.

The flap of skin was sewn back to his arm with enough stitches to remind me of my model-train tracks, and he received a transfusion of two pints of blood. Then I spoke to my father's doctor. Or rather he spoke to me.

"Tell your father he's lost a great deal of blood," the doctor said.

"Brilliant man," my father signed, his damaged arm thickly encased in gauze and tape from wrist to elbow.

"My father says thank you for advising him of that fact."

"Tell your father he has to keep his arm dry for the next week, change the dressing twice a day, and apply ointment each time he changes the bandages. I will give you a prescription for the ointment. Tell the druggist you want the ointment in a tube, not in a jar. Tell your father he must drink at least eight glasses of water a day, and he should eat lots of meat, like calves' liver, as he is anemic from the loss of blood."

While the doctor was telling me all this, my father was watching the doctor's mouth with little comprehension but growing anxiety.

"What did the doctor say?" he kept interrupting.

"Later," I answered. "I'll tell you later."

"No! Tell me now! I'm not a child!" My father flung angry signs at me, accompanied by his harsh deaf voice.

The people in the hospital corridor stared with rude fascination at my father and his excited hand-signing. Others looked on in disgust and cringed at his screeching deaf voice, which reverberated down the hallway, stopping people in their tracks.

With my brother at my side, I wanted to shout at them, *What are you looking at? We're not freaks.*

My father saw my eyes drift away from his and understood what he read in my face, my shame and anger, guilt, and embarrassment.

"Pay no attention to the hearing people," he fairly shouted at me in sign. "They are stupid. They don't know better. They don't know our deaf ways."

As I began to explain to my father what the doctor had said, the doctor interrupted me, saying, "I'm quite busy. I can't spend more time with your father. Tell him—"

My father pulled my arm. *"What is the doctor saying?"* His signs squeaked like chalk across the blackboard of my mind.

I begged the doctor to be patient with my father. I asked my father to be patient with me. I assured my brother that our father would be all right. And my head began to throb with a headache.

Eventually I transmitted all the necessary instructions from the doctor to my father, my father's many questions to the doctor, and the doctor's abrupt answers to my father in highly edited form.

At last my father was satisfied and we went home.

I sat between my father and my brother in the subway car, the three of us leaning into each other, away from the other passengers. I answered as best I could the additional questions that occurred to my father. My brother had no questions to ask. He was simply grateful to be going home.

Suddenly my father took me in his arms and kissed my face. "I'm sorry I need you to be my voice in the hearing world. Especially when there is a big emergency." He looked deeply into my eyes and told me he loved me and was proud of me this day.

His sign for *proud* was expansive. His thumb rose against his chest, tracing a passage from waist to neck, while his chest expanded with exaggerated pride.

After what seemed an eternity, we were home. When my father rang the bell, triggering the bulb inside the apartment that announced our arrival in flashing lights, my mother threw open the door. She was frantic, a look of naked fear spread across her face. She had no idea what had happened to her family. She had arrived home to an empty apartment, seen the blood, and realized there had been a terrible accident. But who was hurt? Who had shed so much blood? And where were we? She did not know. She had had no one to ask. She had no phone, nor any way of using it if she had one, and we had left in too much of a panic for me to have thought about writing her a note.

At the sight of my father my mother's fear dissolved into such profound relief that it nearly broke my heart. An explosion of joy burst across her face, and she made sounds I had never heard her make before: sounds from her heart. Paying no attention to his bandages, she flung herself into his arms. With his damaged arm, my father held her close, burying his face in her hair. My brother and I were completely ignored.

As young as I was, I understood what her reaction meant: she had not, after all, lost her only partner in silence in this alien hearing world. And even at that early age the thought came to me: *What would it be like if one of them died and the other had to go on living? How could they endure the loss?*

I knew deep down that in some way I had aged this day, and that I now understood the isolated world of my deaf father and mother as I never had before.

21
My Brother's Keeper

Shortly after his diagnosis of epilepsy, my brother was put on a daily dose of phenobarbital, which impeded his ability to function both physically and mentally. Phenobarbital was such a powerful drug that the Nazis had used high doses of it to kill children born with diseases and deformities that kept them from meeting the so-called standards of the Aryan race. Of course, we didn't know that during the years it was being administered to my brother. But we could see, only too clearly, that his daily dose often left him confused, and so lethargic that he sometimes appeared to be sleepwalking.

Nonetheless, he was never held back in school. This, of course, created many problems. Since he had no way under the circumstances to keep up with his schoolwork, on many occasions his teachers sent him home early with a handwritten note requesting that my father come in for a conference.

These meetings meant that my father had to get a half-day off from work, and that I had to get permission to skip a half-day of school. The former was a hardship, the latter an embarrassment. Prior to each of these school meetings, my father insisted that we take my brother in to meet his doctor, so as to get a professional opinion of his ability to do the work.

During these meetings my role as interpreter for my father was put to the maximum test. At the doctor's office I had to interpret for my father the doctor's assessment of what could be expected of my brother, and the medical reasons for those expectations. Then I had to interpret for the doctor the questions my father wanted to ask in response. The resulting delays in their communication soon became frustrating for both of them.

To compound the difficulties of this linguistic Gordian knot, the doctor's nurse kept popping in to breathlessly announce that the waiting room was filled to capacity and that the doctor's patients were threatening to find another doctor, one who was not so busy. Of course, I had to interpret this for my father as well.

"So tell her to tell those idiots to get another doctor," my father instructed me. Whether he was serious or not, I never knew. I mouthed some unintelligible but bland nonsense in the general direction of the nurse as she turned and left the office, hoping my father couldn't read my lips.

And all the while my brother would be looking at me beseechingly, waiting for me to explain what was going on around him and, I thought, to speak up for him. In these situations, with both the doctor and my father clamoring for my attention and my translations, I was hard-pressed to take the time to give my brother the reassurance that he so badly needed.

As I grew older, my resentment of my brother's dependence on me faded. I felt sorry for him—for the state of near helplessness to which the epilepsy and the treatment for it had reduced him, oscillating between seizure and recovery, and for the way he tried so hard to be just like the other kids on our street. But the epilepsy did gradually loosen its grip on him, until, at about the time he turned ten, his epileptic seizures stopped, just as suddenly and inexplicably as they had begun. He was at last relieved of his daily torture: the bruises from his falls, the swollen, bitten tongue that filled his mouth, the chipped teeth, and the nausea and headaches that lasted for hours.

Once he was able to go off most of his medications, he gained some confidence and embarked on what would become his childhood passion: roller-skating. Tentatively, then with growing trust in his newfound abilities, he went on skating excursions around our neighborhood. At first he could barely navigate on his wobbly ankles the length of our block. Eventually, with dogged determination, he could skate around our block—up Ninth Street to Avenue P, around the corner, down Tenth Street to Stillwell Avenue, and back to our building on Ninth Street. In time he would, with ever-increasing skill, be able to skate from our block to Coney Island, three miles away, and then back again. At the meetings with our family doctor, and then with my brother's teachers, I would offer this newfound skill, and the discipline that

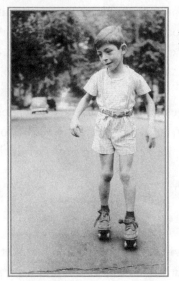

Irwin on his roller skates

made it possible, as an indication that he could also keep up with his schoolwork.

The doctor visits always proceeded in the same way. After talking to all of us and doing seemingly endless tests on my brother to ascertain his cognitive abilities, the doctor invariably instructed me: "Tell your father that with extra attention your brother can at least keep up with his grade level."

After each such visit to the doctor we would go to my brother's school, where I would resume the back-and-forthing of my role as translator. Round after round of meetings would ensue, and at each meeting a teacher would ask the foundational questions: "Who will be responsible for helping the boy keep up with his classmates?" Silence. Much looking at one another. Much sage nodding of heads. "Who will be providing the extra hours of work explaining the boy's homework to him?" Continued silence. Eye-avoiding looks. Heads bobbing. "And who will be monitoring his progress on a daily basis?"

I interpreted each of the teacher's questions for my father.

"Well?" the teacher would demand, looking at my father for the first time during this protracted conversation. Normally, in these types of interactions, the hearing person never looked at my father but rather at me. As for my father, to them he might as well have been a tree stump.

"Well . . ." my father hesitantly signed, staring helplessly back at the teacher. My brother, knowing that he was the focus of this back-and-forth exercise, looked at them both, while they in turn looked back at him.

Then, as one, they all looked at me.

*H*ide-and-seek was a wildly popular Brooklyn street game that we kids played with youthful abandon and enduring passion. Its rules were simple. To begin the game, one unlucky person was designated It. This kid, so identified, would remain It until he (girls had no interest in this game) succeeded in tagging another unlucky kid, while shouting, "You're It." And so the game continued, with successive kids becoming It, until we were too tired or bored to play any longer.

This simple street game, requiring no bat, glove, ball, or any other special equipment, operated on the principle of tension and release—tension at being singled out as It, and the anticipated release of transferring that role to someone else. The appeal resided in the fact that there always *was* someone else.

As a child playing with my friends on my Brooklyn block, I loved this game. When my turn came, I didn't mind at all the brief period during which I played the role of It.

But as the same child living upstairs in apartment 3A, I deeply resented that I was always and eternally It. My father's use of me in certain situations was akin to his use of a tool selected with care from his carpenter's toolbox. In 3A there would never be anyone else I could transfer that role to by the simple expedient of a tag.

22
Dad, Jackie, and Me

It was the golden summer of 1947. Now that I had turned fourteen, my father gave me a belated birthday present, one that I had dreamed about but never thought I would see. Coming home from work one night, a triumphant expression on his face, he held up two baseball tickets.

Sign was unnecessary.

My father had never played sports as a boy and, with the exception of boxing, didn't seem to have much interest as an adult. But he had loved the Brooklyn Dodgers ever since they signed Jackie Robinson earlier that year. Jackie Robinson was a black man and a great athlete. It was a new world now, and a black man was playing first base for our home team. Who would have thought it possible?

My father put down the paper and handed me the precious pair of thick cardboard tickets that announced in black bold letters, "Brooklyn Dodgers vs. St. Louis Cardinals." We fans in Brooklyn hated the Cards with such enduring passion, the words might as well have been "Brooklyn Goes to War."

My father took up a batter's stance and wagged an invisible bat menacingly over his shoulder, his eyes squinting, the better to see the arrival over the plate of an invisible spinning baseball that he appeared to be completely capable of smashing out of the park.

I was puzzled. I simply could not fathom my father's sudden interest in Jackie Robinson. I knew my father's history well, as he enjoyed telling me stories of when he was a boy my age. As a deaf boy in a deaf residential military academy at the turn of the last century, he had had few opportunities for play of any kind, including sports. First he had had to learn discipline, for in those days deaf children were thought by their hearing teachers to be ungovernable animals. Then he had to be taught the basics of reading and writing—an arduous process for the teachers, and a grueling one for the pupils. Play was a luxury available only to the hearing kids, the teachers at his school said. The deaf would have to spend every minute of their young lives trying to keep up, since they would always be behind—deaf in a hearing world.

Baffled as I was by my father's sudden desire to go to a baseball game, I certainly didn't let it get in the way of my own excitement. I had never been to Ebbets Field and had never seen the Dodgers play. This was going to be a great event in my life.

I was an overnight sensation on my block when I showed my friends—but did not allow them to touch—the two baseball tickets. I slept with those two tickets under my pillow every night and never let them out of my sight during daylight hours.

Finally the big day arrived. I will never forget the look of the entrance to Ebbets Field, the elegant curve of the rotunda that drew us into that hallowed place. Once we passed through the clacking wooden turnstile, clutching our ticket stubs for dear life, we ascended with the excited mob up the dimly lit stone ramp beneath the towering concrete ceiling, out a small doorway, and into an arena overlooking a field of impossibly green grass. Down below us the grassy expanse was bisected by perfectly groomed brown base paths, bordered by strictly drawn powdered white lines stretching into infinity, all of it sparkling like a polished diamond in soft summer sunlight.

So *this* is what it looks like in real life, I thought.

Like every other kid in Brooklyn, I listened on the radio to Red Barber announce every single Dodger game of the season. Indeed, you could not walk down my block without hearing the Old Redhead calling out "balls" and "strikes" from every open window. I now realized that the images I had conjured up in my mind's eye from listening to the radio were little more than black and white silhouettes, while *this* magnificent sight was in living Technicolor.

Our seats were perfect, box seats right on the first-base line, not fifty feet from Jackie Robinson. Jackie made his presence known soon after the umpire called, "Play ball!" He smacked a double off the left-field wall, sending the runner home for the first run of the day.

The game quickly turned into a pitching duel. But late in the game the Cards tied the score. Inning after inning, play after play, my father showered me with questions. With one eye on the action and the other on my father, I tried my best to describe, in abbreviated signs, the finer points of the game. Up until that time I had never actually seen a professional baseball game, but having listened to Red Barber I felt I was an expert.

Then the unthinkable happened. A Cardinal batter, racing down the first-base line in an impossible attempt to beat out a ground ball, intentionally spiked Jackie's leg, long after the ball had arrived in his glove.

Twenty-six thousand Brooklyn fans leaped to their feet, and the stands erupted in protest. Cries of outrage poured from twenty-six thousand mouths, swirled up the aisles, bounced off the girders, and reverberated against the roof.

"JACKIEE! JACKIEE! JACKIEE!" they screamed.

My father's shouts of "AH-GHEE! AH-GHEE! AH-GHEE!" went unheard in the Niagara of sound.

Jackie Robinson just stood there on first base, bright red blood streaming down his leg, with a face that looked as if it had been carved in black marble.

Later that day Jackie got another hit off the Cardinal pitcher, and the fans went nuts.

"JACKIEE! JACKIEE! JACKIEE!"

"AH-GHEE! AH-GHEE! AH-GHEE!"

This time the fans in the neighboring seats looked at my father. He must surely have been aware of their stares, but he kept his eyes locked on Jackie, who was beginning to edge off second base. I looked at my feet.

On the subway ride home my father signed, "I am a deaf man in a hearing world. All the time I must show hearing people that I am a man as well. A man as good as them. Maybe even better."

The subway car was packed. As usual, people in the car stared at my father with mixed looks of curiosity, shock, and even revulsion. I paid no attention to them as I watched his hands.

"Jackie Robinson is a black man in the white man's baseball world. All the time he must show white people that he is a man. A man as good as them. Maybe even better. No matter that his skin is a black color. The color of his skin is not important. Only what Jackie does on the ball field is important."

Just when I thought my father had finished speaking, his hands spoke to me sorrowfully. "Very hard for a deaf man. Very hard for a black man. Must fight all the time. No rest. *Never*. Sad."

My father didn't sign another word. He just stared into the eyes of the subway riders looking rudely at him, until they sheepishly broke off eye contact—every last one of them.

We went to many more home games during that summer of 1947. Somehow my father always got box-seat tickets along the first-base line. To this day I can hear with perfect clarity his delighted cries of "AH-GHEE! AH-GHEE! AH-GHEE!" Cries that seemed to come straight from his heart.

23
Silent Snow

*O*ne night in December, as 1947 was drawing to a close, I was awakened by a profound silence, a total absence of sound of any kind. It was as if my bedroom had been smothered by a giant down-filled pillow. It was a silence that had weight. A silence that filled our small apartment as completely as water fills a fish tank.

As we lived in a third-floor apartment in Brooklyn, there was *always* noise, night and day. During daylight hours, the sounds of children playing, and adults gossiping and arguing and complaining, drifted up to my open bedroom window. At night, the children safely in bed, the adults hit the street below my window to continue their gossiping and arguing and complaining in their distinctive Brooklyn voices. But not this night. As my brother slept on, unaware, I went to my window and saw the most remarkable sight: an impenetrable white wall of falling snow. Some twenty hours later it would be recorded as the greatest snowfall in the history of Brooklyn, exceeding even the legendary record-setting "Blizzard of 1888" by over five inches. (Like all records, my childhood "blizzard" would later be eclipsed. It would happen some fifty-nine years later, though only by half an inch.)

In that deep silence, I heard my father muttering in his sleep. Looking into his room, I saw him tossing and turning in great agitation while locked in a dream that would not let him go. His hands were signing his dream.

The next morning, all of us kept at home by the new-fallen snow, I asked him if he dreamed in sign.

"I don't know," he said. "I never thought to wonder."

"Do you think in sign?" I asked.

"I'm not sure," he answered. "All my thinking comes at once. Sometime I see a complete picture in my head."

Then he hesitated. "Wait. That's not all true. Sometimes I think about a problem with sign pictures. Also, sometimes I talk out my thinking to myself with my hands. My language is in my hands. My memories are in my hands. All my thinking is in my hands."

Then my father's hands told me a story:

"When I was a young man in the Depression, I knew a deaf boy who worked in a dangerous factory. He had no choice. He had to bring his family some money to buy food to eat. There were many people in his family, and his father was dead, so the boy had to be the father.

"The deaf boy worked six days a week, twelve hours a day. He got very tired. One day he was so tired, he paid no close attention to the machine he was working on, and the machine took off the fingers of his right hand. All the fingers. After his hand healed, the deaf boy lost his language. He could only talk with one hand. Deaf people did not clearly understand him. Very sad. Now I have nightmares of this bad thing happening to me."

My father stopped signing and stared at his hands with a look of terror on his face.

"How would I talk if such a terrible thing happened to me?" he signed. "My language is in my hands. How would I tell of my love for my beautiful Sarah? And if I had no hands, how would I touch and hold my boys?"

Then he looked out the window at the accumulated snow piled deeply in front of our apartment house. Nothing was moving on our block. Nothing was visible: no blacktop street, no sewers, no curb, no fire hydrant, no iron picket fence, no garbage cans, no stoop, no cars. But here and there in the vast whiteness were occasional humps in the snow blanket, shadowy shapes that suggested what lay beneath.

"Come see what else my hands can do," he signed, grabbing a snow shovel with one hand and my sled in the other. I took my brother's hand, and our father marched us out of our apartment, down the stairs, and out into what seemed, to my brother and me, the North Pole.

24
Pigskin Dreams

*W*hen I turned seven, my father bought me an authentic Wilson leather football. I could not hold it, as my hand was too small. My mother thought my father a bit premature and told him so. "He will *grow*," he signed to her, his hidden closed right hand appearing ever so slowly from behind his open left covering hand. Rising upward, it grew, spreading wide, flushed with new life. I saw all this in his sign: the petals of a blooming plant unfolding as the stalk of his right arm rose ever higher, seeking the warmth of the sun. Then, so there was no doubt as to how big I'd be one day, he held his right hand palm down at his waist, and slowly raised it until it was over his head—and he smiled.

Watching my father's sign, I tried to imagine myself someday as strong as he was and even taller. That, I thought, could not be possible.

I was more fascinated by my father's signs than I was with the large clumsy object, now forgotten, that he had placed into my hands.

My father wanted desperately for me to have the childhood he never had—the carefree joy of his brother and sisters at play, which he'd watched from afar.

I grew. And as I grew, my father encouraged me to play the various street games of our block, the same games that were played on every block and in every neighborhood of Brooklyn.

Unlike my friends' fathers, who were usually too tired after a day's work or too preoccupied with the lengthening reach of the Depression, my father was an avid and in time a knowledgeable observer of these street games. And he was my greatest fan. As my friends and I played, he would stand on the curb, which was the sideline of our football field and the third-base line of our stickball games. Our "playing field" was not covered in the soft green grass of a real football field but in black unyielding macadam, interrupted by the occasional cast-iron manhole cover. All in all, it was a most inhospitable surface upon which to slide or fall.

And yet I would fall, and I would slide. Each fall and slide was accompanied by my father's deaf voice shouting encouragement. "Great catch!" "You're safe!" Though my friends could make no sense of these harsh sounds, I understood them, and they were the unremarked-upon accompaniment to many of our games.

One memorable day, while reaching for a winning touchdown pass, I ran into a parked car. My last conscious thought was that I had my man beat. I woke up in Coney Island Hospital. The first person I saw was my father sitting beside my bed. "You scored," he signed. Then he added, "Now what the heck will we tell Mother?"

*O*n a late-summer day when I had just turned sixteen, I reported for football tryouts, which were held on our high school football field. The field, like our school, was new—so new that it lacked even a single blade of grass. I would shortly discover that it did not lack other objects, most noticeably stones. I would further observe that those stones, randomly seeded, were uniformly hard. But I figured this field could not be any harder than the macadam on which I had learned to play the game.

The coach presiding over the tryouts was Harry Ostro, who had served with the 101st Airborne in World War II. Ostro had been a paratrooper in the largest airborne battle in history, Operation Market Garden, which was immortalized some thirty years later in the movie *A Bridge Too Far*. After successfully leading his platoon inside enemy lines, Ostro had been seriously wounded. But all I knew about him at the time, and only because it was all too visible, was that he had a metal plate in his head—something he never spoke about. The coach was, then and now, the toughest man I ever met. (He still pumps out fifty push-ups a day, having recently turned ninety-two.) The coach didn't talk, he growled.

I made the squad that day—not for my negligible skills, but for my ability to survive the grueling physical and mental demands he imposed on us—and spent the next three months in mortal fear. Like my teammates, I never feared the opposing team. It was our coach we feared.

My father came to every game. Although I rode the bench, rarely seeing any action, he could not be dissuaded from coming. In rain or shine, sleet, and once in a driving early-season snowstorm, he was there. Sitting on the bench, my back turned to the stands, I couldn't see my father, but I could hear his guttural voice as it cut through the shouts of the other spectators.

High school was a new world for me. My fellow students had rarely if ever seen a deaf man before, and I had dreaded the prospect of watching them stiffen, as people almost invariably did, at the strange sound of my father's voice. My teammates, however, soon grew accustomed to my father, just as my friends on the block had. And they came to appreciate him for being such a loyal fan of our team.

Football was my passport to normalcy in high school. At that age especially, kids have a strong desire to fit in, to be like the others, to be part of the crowd, and as the child of deaf parents, I yearned more than most to hide behind a shield of normalcy. Because of football, I ceased to be known as the deaf man's son; instead I was known as a football player.

When my first season ended and I was awarded a football letter, my mother sewed it onto my varsity sweater. I wore that sweater until it was in tatters.

The following year I grew two inches and added twenty pounds to my previously scrawny frame. I had matured enough for my coach to use me in games more frequently. At least, he reasoned, I wouldn't be killed.

My father came to every game, as usual. Now we would spend the evening after the contest analyzing the good and bad plays. My father caught on fast, becoming an astute student of football. But to describe the nuances of the game, we had to teach ourselves a whole new vocabulary of signs.

The night before the final game of that season, unbeknownst to us, our star tailback fell down a flight of stairs and landed, right hand extended, on a broken milk bottle. The next afternoon he showed up for the game—at the field of our archrivals, New Utrecht High School—with his arm heavily bandaged. He could not suit up. The team was in a state of shock. Joe Darienzo was a senior. This was to be his last game. He was Brooklyn's best tailback and the leader of our team. We all sat there in the locker room prior to the opening kickoff, dejected and with a sense of impending doom.

The coach stood with his arm draped over Joe's shoulder and addressed the team.

"Men, this is the most important game of the season."

We knew that.

"Joe wanted more than anything to play this game. But he can't."

We knew that.

"Joe is an important part of this team. But it is the *team* that wins or loses, not any single man."

We knew that.

"As a *team*, we can win this game today."

We weren't at all sure of that.

Then he told us that I would start in Joe's place.

That I hadn't known. Nor had the team or my father. But when my father saw me in the backfield behind the center on the very first play, he knew that this would be a memorable game. And he began to dream up new football signs, since we would have much to discuss that evening.

How much, I had no idea as I stood in a daze waiting to receive the opening hike. Our center was looking back at me, upside down between his legs, with obvious skepticism on his face. His look did little to reassure me. The rest of the game passed in a blur. The only solid memory I have is being yelled at. The coach yelled at me. Joe, overcoat slung over his shoulder, his arm in a sling, ranging up and down the sidelines, yelled at me. My father, who had been given a sideline pass for the game, yelled at me, as he relentlessly recorded my every boneheaded mistake on his wind-up movie camera.

Every pass I threw was a picture-perfect spiral . . . right into the hands of a waiting defensive receiver. Every run I made was stopped at the line of scrimmage. Every inept hand-off to another backfield man I attempted was fumbled.

However, my teammates played an exemplary game, more than making up for my mistakes. In the final quarter we were tied. In the waning minutes our coach came up with a desperation play, an all-or-nothing shot at winning. It was based on the assumption that, given my pathetic performance all that long afternoon, nobody on the opposing team would be paying me much attention. As a threat, I was about as dangerous as our head cheerleader. So no one would wonder why the hike from center would go not to me, as was normal, but to our fullback, who was to my right. Exaggerating the fact that I was empty-handed, I veered to the left. (Being adept at sign language, I was an excellent mime and finally I had a role on this miserable afternoon that I could fill.) Meanwhile, the fullback made a big show of handing the ball off to Tommy La Spada, our shifty wingback, who was headed in the other direction. While this dumb show was playing itself out in the backfield, our linemen went into a choreographed ballet, feinting this way and that, confusing not only the opposing team but themselves as well.

In the midst of all the hullabaloo, with studied nonchalance I drifted back to my right, and Tommy, coming from the other direction, handed the ball to me with such deft sleight-of-hand that the oncoming defensive end missed the move. One look at the fierce expression on his face, and Tommy realized that the end was setting himself up to crush him to the ground. Tommy, although tough as nails, was one of the smallest members of the team—and he was no fool. I heard him scream, *"I don't have the ball!"* That was a clarion call for me to get out of there fast.

Our cartoon play was so successful that no one now was watching me—and I ran for my life down the right sideline, unnoticed and untouched, and scored a touchdown. We had won the game, just as our coach had said. The crowd went wild. Through all the outpouring of sound, I could clearly make out my father's harsh, whooping voice.

That evening my father laughingly taught me the strangest signs I would ever learn in my lifetime.

25

Exodus

My senior year in high school, I was offered a football scholarship to Brandeis University, a brand-new school in New England that had sophomore, junior, and senior classes but needed a freshman class. It also needed football players who would be willing to take the chance of going to a school that wouldn't even be eligible for accreditation for another two years.

I had also been offered a football scholarship to NYU—but their campus was in the Bronx, and if I accepted that offer, it would mean continuing to live at home and commuting to school by subway. I never considered it for a moment.

My father was ecstatic. I would be the first on either side of my family to go to college.

"You must look like a college man," he signed. "I don't want them to think you're a yokel from the sticks." Brooklyn? The *sticks*? I didn't argue. My going to college was going to be as exciting an experience for him as it would be for me. And I wouldn't deny him the pleasure of dressing me up like a college man. Our once-a-year trips to Mr. Bloomingdale and Mr. R. and H. Macy became an almost weekly ritual the summer after my senior year in high school. Clutching photographs of college men torn out of magazines in his hand, my father scoured the racks of suits to find those that would make me look the part, and—perhaps more important—would last for four years.

One day in early August my father accompanied me, newly bought suitcase in hand, to Grand Central Station, where I would catch the train to Boston. I was dressed in a heavy wool tweed suit. It was about ninety degrees in the station. I did not sign one word of complaint. As the conductor shouted "All aboard!" my father looked me over one last time and signed, "You look like a college man for sure." Then he added, "I'll see you soon." Little did I know how true that would be. For the next four years my father came to almost every home game we played, always carrying a heavy CARE package that my mother had lovingly prepared all that week.

Stepping onto the train that day, I took the final step, the step from my parents' deaf world, so familiar yet so foreign, to my own world, the world of the hearing.

Thereafter, when I was with my parents, I would be only a visitor to their world of eternal silence. It had been, for me, a world of great beauty filled with limitless love and, God help me, frequent shame. It had also been a difficult world in which a child had had to play the role of an adult.

The sign for *responsibility* is a dramatic one and leaves little room for doubt as to its meaning. It was one of the first signs my father taught me. He would place both hands, fingertips relentlessly pressing downward, on his right shoulder. His shoulder would slump, as if bearing a great burden, and his face would assume a look of patient endurance. This was what was always expected of me: to be responsible—for my father and his needs, and then when my brother became sick, for my brother, too. There were times when I found this burden crushing, and those were the days when I would rush from my apartment to the roof of our building and hide for hours on end.

Now as I sat on the cushioned seat of the railroad car directly over the iron wheels that relentlessly carried me away, with each revolution, from the only home I had ever known, I felt a lifting of this ever-present burden of responsibility. From now on I would not be responsible for my father or my brother. They would have to manage for themselves.

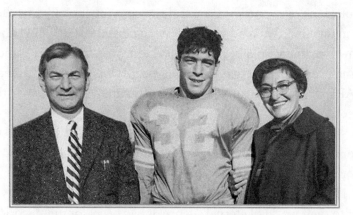

My mother and father after a football game
at Brandeis University, 1951. We won.

My sense of relief, however, was diluted by an inexplicable sense of loss. It had never occurred to me that I would feel that way.

26

The Duke of Coney Island

My uncle David was my mother's favorite of her three brothers. "He is a magician, a sorcerer," she always said of this brother, who was one year younger than she. David was a sorcerer to my mother because, with a wink of his devilish brown eyes, he could transform her sadness into joy. He treated her deafness with remarkable nonchalance. Where every other member of her family made my mother feel different, David acted as if her deafness were nothing more important, or significant, than the color of her eyes or the texture of her hair.

Everyone in my mother's family, as well as all of his many friends, called David "the Duke of Coney Island." This was in acknowledgment of his suave manner, his elegant clothes, and the way he managed to get by in such high style with no steady job.

David and my mother were both splendid swimmers. With the sun rising over the beach at Coney Island, holding hands and laughing, they would launch themselves into the Atlantic Ocean and swim until they were out of sight. My mother's powerful, tanned arms would cleave the water, and she and her white bathing cap would grow ever smaller until, at the edge of the horizon, she and David disappeared.

I always waited patiently on the shore, my father and brother at my side. My father, who was great with his hands, helped us build the most intricate and fantastic sand castles, as we sat and waited for my mother to emerge from the sea.

My father never joined my mother in the water, as he could barely swim three consecutive strokes without stopping to gasp for air. But before diving in himself, David always made a show of grabbing my father's arm and trying to drag him into the water, while my brother took the other arm and, digging his toes into the sand, pulled in the other direction. This was just a game they played—there was no way my father would go into the ocean with David. "I grew up in the Bronx," my father would explain, if anyone wondered why he remained on shore. "No ocean." For him, that explained almost everything, the Bronx being a provincial backwater to cosmopolitan Brooklyn, with its magnificent stone bridge at one end and the great Atlantic Ocean washing up on the beach at the other.

Eventually, with the sun now high in the sky, I would spot a white dot bobbing between the swells. As I watched, the dot became my mother, her strong brown arms cutting through the water as she swam to shore, followed closely by David.

Sometimes she caught me unawares. Riding an incoming wave like a porpoise, she would slither from the surf, a sea creature, and take my sun-warmed body into her icy-wet embrace.

"Where did you go?" I always asked.

"Ireland," she finger-spelled, with a straight face. "Very green."

In addition to being a great swimmer and a sorcerer, David was a wizard. He could do magic tricks—wondrous, surpassingly amazing sleight-of-hand stunts that left me gasping.

Beginning when I turned six, he began the ritual of pulling objects from my ear on every birthday. That first year it was a penny. When I turned seven, it was a nickel. At eight, he produced a dime from the depths of my ear. And at nine, a quarter. The following year it was a half-dollar.

The year I turned eleven, my uncle David, after much hocus-pocus, rolled up the sleeve of his right arm and, with great exaggeration, displayed his empty hand under my nose. Wiggling the five digits in the air, he proceeded with infinite slowness to curl his middle finger, then the finger to its left, and finally his pinky into a ball. With the remaining forefinger and thumb, he formed a pincered claw.

Slowly he moved the claw to my ear, then into my ear, and with much grunting and twisting, he extracted a gleaming uncirculated silver dollar. It was magnificent.

Placing the silver dollar on its edge, with a deft twist of his fingers he set it spinning on a nearby surface. "This coin reminds me of you," he said before the coin came to a stop. I nodded solemnly, not having a clue as to his meaning.

Many years later, when we were both living in Los Angeles, I was riding in a car with my uncle when he asked me if I remembered my eleventh birthday and the silver dollar he had pulled from my ear.

He then explained what he had meant to say to me that day when he had set the coin spinning. As a child, David said, I always seemed to him to be two sides of the same coin, both one thing and its opposite. I was cleaved into two parts, half hearing, half deaf, forever joined together. And he had observed, very astutely, that I vacillated and vibrated between the child that I was in years and the adult I was forced to be in thought and action. When he looked at me, he saw that I stood at the crossroads of sound and silence, of childhood and adulthood, and that I would have to struggle to find my own way.

With his explanation I realized, perhaps as never before, how hard I had fought, all of my young life, to break free from my father's eternal need of me. It was a struggle that I waged to assert my independence, my very right to be a child. But it was a struggle I fought with one small hand tied behind my back, since I could not let my father think for even one moment that I was abandoning him and the overpowering burden of his deafness.

On that long ride I took with my uncle, across Mulholland, over the Sepulveda Pass, and down into the Valley, heading toward his apartment, I thought about the other side of my childhood's equation: my mother's need of me. As her firstborn hearing son, I met a need in her that was of an exclusively practical, utilitarian nature. Unlike my father, she used me only for the nuts and bolts of her everyday forced interactions with the hearing world: *What is the price of this? The availability of that?*

Perhaps the differences between my mother and father had to do with the fact that my mother had been deafened as an infant. She had no memory of sound, which for her was intangible, an abstraction, merely an idea. But my father, unlike my mother, had been deafened later in life. Until the age of three he could hear. Somewhere, buried in the folds of his brain, was the memory of sound. That memory, elusive, fragmentary, would not release him. It hovered somewhere always on the horizon of his consciousness. Through me he would try to find it, to tease it into being. And he looked to me to provide the clues.

My father needed me to help him remember sound. To understand sound itself. The very essence of sound. Sound in all its guises. Sound in all its permutations. The shape and physicality of sound. Even the color of sound. Or as a synesthete might, the sound of color.

He struggled all of my young life to fathom spoken speech. How could it be that speech emerged from the mouth of the hearing invisible, yet had substance? How did sound travel invisibly through the equally invisible air to enter the hearing ear, where it rushed over and caressed a billion tiny hairs deep in the ear canal, like sea grass waving tremulously to the unheard tune of invisible currents?

And the biggest mystery of all: How did the vibrations transmit sound to the mind, where it was *heard*?

His questions began when I was six years old. I could never answer them satisfactorily, and they would not cease until I left his deaf world forever, twelve years later, college-bound.

Once I was no longer a trusted resident of his world, merely a visitor, something changed between us and his questions ceased. Many years later I realized that with my departure, his unquenchable quest for the understanding of sound had ended; he had asked no more questions of me.

To this day, when I think of my father, and I recall so vividly the intensity of my childhood, I remember my uncle David's birthday gift: the silver dollar.

Oh, how I wish I had saved it. I would set it spinning. What would it tell me now?

27
Death, a Stranger

I knew of death early and late.

When I was six years old, I saw a man standing on the edge of an apartment house roof on my block. He had been standing there for some time, motionless, on the low brick wall that was the dividing line between the tar-papered, gravel-covered roof to his back and the air over Brooklyn at his feet. Staring straight ahead, he could see the Atlantic Ocean at Coney Island. Looking down, he could see the concrete sidewalk of West Ninth Street, six floors below his feet.

I watched, hypnotized, in a state of incomprehension, alongside a group of neighbors at the curb directly across the street from the building. We stood there, looking up at him, as he poured gasoline over his head and shoulders and, in one incandescent instant, lit a match and burst into flame.

As I watched in stunned disbelief, not really understanding what my eyes were telling my brain, he calmly stepped off the roof in a ball of fire. Trailing sparks and bits of flaming clothing, he fell directly onto the low iron picket fence that fronted the building. The fence buckled at the impact of his falling body. He lay impaled on a pike of the picket fence, smoldering, his clothing turning to ash as the green paint on the fence blistered, then bubbled away. For weeks afterward I would come across bits of charred fabric lying around the building.

The man was a stranger. He had come to our block to die. My father could not tell me why. For once, his hands were silent.

Many years later, when I was an army paratrooper with the 82nd Airborne Division, my father and mother came down to visit me at Fort Bragg, near Fayetteville, North Carolina, where I was stationed. And, of course, my father had timed their visit to coincide with a mass parachute jump, which is always an impressive sight. As wave after wave of C-119s took off from Pope Air Force Base, each wave of planes flew at an altitude barely fifty feet above the preceding wave, leaving just enough space between them that their propellers would not chew up the jumpers hanging in the air in front of them. In stately formation they passed over the three-mile-long sandy drop zone, thousands of parachutists jumping out the twin doors. The sky was filled, horizon to horizon, with slowly descending white silk petals. But one of those parachutists got into trouble. His static line had become entangled with the shoulder strap on his parachute.

The soldier dangled at the end of the canvas line for hours, as the crew, the copilot, and jumpmaster vainly attempted to pull him back into the plane, against the backstream of the twin propellers. It was useless, as the pressure of the turbulent air created by the backdraft of the propellers was simply too powerful a force to overcome.

Once the plane had burned up all its fuel flying in circles for hours, a layer of foam was sprayed on the runway and the plane was forced to land. As it rolled down the runway, the body trailed behind and bounced up and down in the foam.

It was later reported that the soldier had been unconscious when the plane touched down. But we all knew that was bull.

That evening my father talked about death. This was strange, because my father had never brought up the subject before. Even when his father died and we went to his funeral in the Bronx, my father had barely signed a thought to me. And when his mother had died, he cried but did not talk.

But during dinner that night he talked of death. The sign for death is one of the most poignant of signs, and one of the most descriptive in its abrupt visual expressiveness. It leaves no doubt as to its meaning. My father, in expressing his feelings about death and dying that night, constantly held his open hands in front of him, right palm down, death, left palm up, life. In that position, he stared at them thoughtfully and then reversed them.

"Death," he signed, "is a stranger. Just like the stranger who came to our street to die."

Later, much later, in another season, my father spent his last day on earth in the same hospital in Coney Island where I was born. There was not one person around him to whom he could express his resignation, his regrets, or his fears in his own language.

It has been twenty-nine years since my father died, alone, in a hospital ward in Brooklyn, filled with strangers who could not speak to him and who could not read his hands. If he had had the strength to do so, he would surely have left his bed and walked the few feet to a window of the ward to look out on the sandy beach of Coney Island, where fifty years previously he had first seen the dark-haired laughing deaf girl who would become his wife.

My mother and I had been with him all that day (my brother, at the time, was working in Virginia), and we had just gone out to get something to eat. My mother had signed as she left his bedside, "We'll be *right* back." When we returned to his room, barely an hour after we left him, his bed was empty and had been neatly remade.

No one on the floor could tell us where my father was.

"Try the morgue," one nurse advised over her shoulder as she rushed about.

With my frantic mother at my side, we descended in the elevator to the basement morgue.

Exiting the elevator, we found ourselves in a dimly lit circular lobby empty of any living people—but filled end to end with sheet-covered gurneys. My mother jackknifed into herself and stayed closed as if she would never open again. I held her to me.

Unfolding finally, she shook me off and went to the first gurney. She lifted the sheet, glanced at the face beneath, and moved on. From gurney to gurney she repeated the process: lift a corner of the sheet, take a quick look, and move on. Eventually, she stopped moving on, and flung herself across the cold, still body of my dead father.

At the entrance to the Brooklyn cemetery where my father was to be buried, a short line of Orthodox Jewish men stood forlornly along the roadside in the lightly falling rain, hoping to make a few dollars for reciting Kaddish, the traditional Hebrew blessing. My mother asked me to hire one of them to say what she considered to be magic words over her husband's grave.

At my father's open grave, the endless string of words, unheard by my mother and incomprehensible to the rest of us—my brother, my wife, my children, my mother's sister, and my father's two sisters and his brother—droned on endlessly, until I tapped the black-garbed bearded stranger on the shoulder, thanked him, and gave him the agreed-upon payment for his services. Then we stood there, looking at my father's dripping coffin sitting on twin rails, each of us thinking about the man inside, now silent, as we all will be.

$\mathcal{M}$y mother lived another twenty-eight years and remained in relatively good physical health until she was eighty-nine. That year, however, a series of medical problems made it clear she could no longer live on her own.

My brother loved our mother deeply but was still working full-time, now for the City of New York. He agreed that since I was retired and could give her the attention she needed, I would take her with me to Palm Springs (where my wife and I had moved many years before).

No sooner had she settled into her new life with us than she fell to the floor one night and suffered a broken hip—the first of many accidents and illnesses that would slowly but steadily drain her body and her spirit.

During the next six years she would sporadically sign to me, "I want to die!"

"No, you don't," I would say rather inanely. "You have so much to live for." And then I would frantically enumerate all the things I thought she should live for.

My mother would turn away from me, unconvinced.

In frustration one day, I added to the list of things to live for, "*Wait*, I wrote a book."

"You wrote a book?" she signed incredulously. "What's it about?"

"A big snowstorm in Brooklyn," I said, "and a boy who has a dream, and the mother who wakes him with her kiss."

"Sounds interesting. I'll wait for that."

And so my mother lived another six years, waiting first for that book, and then when it was published, and she said, again, "I want to die!" the next book after that one.

Twice a year Irwin would fly out to visit our mother. Her absence from his life was a significant loss. His apartment in New York City had been convenient to hers, and he had been in the habit of visiting her one night during the week, and taking her to a movie and then to dinner on Sundays. With so much time to make up for, my brother found that his biannual ten-day visits seemed to end as soon as they began, which was very hard for him.

Shortly before she died, my mother had been in the hospital on one of her ever more frequently recurring admissions. One morning on my daily visit I found her deeply asleep. Her veined, liver-spotted hands were resting silently at her sides. As I sat by her bed watching, they came alive and began to sign in a language I did not understand. As a boy, I had often seen my mother and father signing their private signs to each other. Signs whose meaning they never shared with me. However, one sign I did recognize: the sign for death.

As I watched my mother, still deeply asleep, signing into the air, I was sure her indecipherable signs were meant for my father. I like to think that she was telling him with her hands, in their private language, that he would not have much longer to wait.

*W*hen we knew my mother had but a week to live, my brother flew out from New York to be at her side. During the week of her dying, my brother and I spent some time talking to each other about our shared experiences as hearing children born to two deaf parents. This was the first time we had ever done so. We spoke often, and late, about our experiences being raised by the people our neighbors at that time called "the deafies in apartment 3A."

Our mother has been dead now for several years, and our father more than thirty, and yet my brother and I still cannot agree on how that shared experience—growing up in apartment 3A with our deaf father and mother, so many years ago—has affected our lives down to this day. We no longer argue about our different impressions of what being deaf meant to them, or about how their being deaf has impacted us; at our age we finally realize that we will never agree.

There is one thing, however, that we do agree on: how much we both loved them, and how terribly we miss them.

I scattered my mother's ashes in the four places I thought she'd like to be remembered, the four compass points of her life.

On a bitterly cold and unseasonably snowy day in early April, I carefully spread some of her ashes, strangely warm and heavy in my hands, in a wide circle over the sands of Coney Island, approximating the circle that the deaf had made in their beach chairs almost eighty years before, when my mother was a beautiful young woman, displaying her perfect young body in a tight-fitting wool bathing suit, her life stretching out into a seemingly distant future. I imagined the depressions in the sand that were made by her small feet. As the wind swirled about me, I watched her bone-white ashes blow off, mingling with the pure white falling snow, to be absorbed forever into the waiting empty sands.

Then I waded into the surf; my legs burned with the shock of the cold water and immediately went numb. As I stood knee-deep in the icy waves that died on the shore and then ebbed away, I released a few more grains of my mother's ashes. They floated off, drawn deeply into the vast ocean, toward Ireland, the same ocean that eighty summers ago she had swum so tirelessly, leaving us behind in the early morning, not returning until the afternoon. I stood on the cold shore remembering how as a boy I would wait at the edge of this ocean until catching sight of her white rubber-capped head bobbing above the waves, her slim nut-brown arms languidly stroking the water, and her strong shoulders sparkling with diamonds of sunlight, as she came straight toward me. Thrashing through the surf, long legs striding against the outgoing tide, she would swoop me up in her arms. I would cling to her, all warm from the sun, my head nuzzling her wet neck, breathing the ends of her cropped matted hair smelling of the deepest ocean.

Later that same day, as the snow continued to fall, I buried some more of my mother's ashes in a small hole I had dug in the ivy-covered mound humped over my father's grave in a cramped Brooklyn cemetery filled with leaning snow-topped headstones. In the profound silence of the empty cemetery, the snow quickly covered the small grave that her ashes rested in, over the larger mound of my father's casket. As I watched, kneeling, head bowed, the snow fell silently, covering everything with its soft blanket.

Back in California, I spread some more of my mother's ashes on the naked stone lip of San Jacinto Mountain, towering ten thousand feet over Palm Springs, where she had lived with me, with occasional pleasure and much resignation, the last six years of her life. In those final years, when our respective roles had been completely reversed, I now the parent, she the child, I came to know my mother, and through her, my childhood, as I never had before. And I recalled the lines of T. S. Eliot: "We shall not cease from exploration / And the end of all our exploring / Will be to arrive where we started / And know the place for the first time."

Finally, in Santa Monica, where my wife and I also have a home (and my mother often visited before she became ill), I spread my mother's ashes in an imaginary line beginning at the base of a solitary cluster of palm trees leaning into each other, which seemed to me to resemble my tight-knit, insular family. The thin trail of ashes continued across the sands of a California beach and ended in the ocean, where I submerged myself in the tumbling surf, letting the sea reclaim from my cupped hand the last few grains.

Now, from the bluff at the foot of my street, a hundred feet above the bustling daily traffic on the Pacific Coast Highway, where no doubt the drivers think of the Dow and not of death, I have an unbroken line of sight over the indwelling palm trees, across the corrugated sand, and into the timeless ocean. From the shoreline, my gaze travels on the broad blue back of the ocean to the blue-gray horizon that bleeds into the gray-blue sky.

Epilogue

*T*here are times, when the house is sleeping, when I remember the smell of my father's body. It is a mixture of many odors, a brisk hint of Old Spice blended with his mug shaving soap, Vitalis, and the sharp odor of the Lava soap he used every night with a stiff brush to clean off the printer's grime that had accumulated under his nails and in the creases of his strong hands.

As a boy, I would sit on the closed toilet seat and watch in fascination as my father scoured his hands until they were pink and fresh.

"My voice is in my hands," he said. "Dirty hands do not speak clearly and with beauty. My hands must be clean, must always be clean."

My father would carefully dry his hands, one strong finger at a time, and then would look down at me with a soft look in his eyes. And his eloquent hands would come to life shaping the air with his perfect love for me.

While I remember, my hands awaken and, independent of me, begin to talk to my father. And as the mists of memory part, I clearly see the hands of my father signing back to me.

*   *   *

*M*any years after the death of my father, when I had the passing thought that I could be an artist, I was studying a book on how to draw the human figure. In the introduction the author extolled the human form as a thing of beauty and infinite complexity, celebrated throughout history by poets and lovers, analyzed and dissected by doctors and architects.

The book then proceeded apace, from a study of The Eyes, The Ears, The Nose, The Mouth, and from there downward.

Eventually, I turned a page, and there was: The Hands.

Displayed on the following pages were marvelous, deceptively simple, pencil line drawings of the human hand in motion.

The accompanying description of the topic began with the sentence "Hands speak a rich language."

Unbidden, my eyes filmed over, and I put down my pencil, and cried.

*   *   *

$\mathcal{M}$any years after the death of my father, when I had the passing thought that I could be an artist, I was studying a book on how to draw the human figure. In the introduction the author extolled the human form as a thing of beauty and infinite complexity, celebrated throughout history by poets and lovers, analyzed and dissected by doctors and architects.

The book then proceeded apace, from a study of The Eyes, The Ears, The Nose, The Mouth, and from there downward.

Eventually, I turned a page, and there was: The Hands.

Displayed on the following pages were marvelous, deceptively simple, pencil line drawings of the human hand in motion.

The accompanying description of the topic began with the sentence "Hands speak a rich language."

Unbidden, my eyes filmed over, and I put down my pencil, and cried.

Epilogue

*T*here are times, when the house is sleeping, when I remember the smell of my father's body. It is a mixture of many odors, a brisk hint of Old Spice blended with his mug shaving soap, Vitalis, and the sharp odor of the Lava soap he used every night with a stiff brush to clean off the printer's grime that had accumulated under his nails and in the creases of his strong hands.

As a boy, I would sit on the closed toilet seat and watch in fascination as my father scoured his hands until they were pink and fresh.

"My voice is in my hands," he said. "Dirty hands do not speak clearly and with beauty. My hands must be clean, must always be clean."

My father would carefully dry his hands, one strong finger at a time, and then would look down at me with a soft look in his eyes. And his eloquent hands would come to life shaping the air with his perfect love for me.

While I remember, my hands awaken and, independent of me, begin to talk to my father. And as the mists of memory part, I clearly see the hands of my father signing back to me.

About the Author

MYRON UHLBERG is the critically acclaimed and award-winning author of a number of children's books. He lives with his wife in Santa Monica and Palm Springs, California.